THE TEMPLE RESET

Detoxing our bodies, renewing the mind,
and reclaiming the spirit

PASTOR BRIAN WRIGHT SR., MSW

THE TEMPLE RESET
Detoxing our bodies, renewing the mind,
and reclaiming the spirit

Copyright 2025 Pastor Brian Wright Sr., MSW

All rights reserved. No part of this publication may be reproduced, distributed or transmitted in any form or by any means, without prior written permission. Unless otherwise identified, scripture quotations are from the King James version of the Bible.

Dreamer Reign Media
P.O. BOX 291354
Port Orange, Florida 32129
www.dreamerreign.com

For Worldwide Distribution
Printed in the U.S.A.

ISBN: 9781952253539

CONTENTS

Foreword 5

Preface 11

Introduction 13

Chapter 1: The Purpose of the Temple Reset 17

Chapter 2: Breaking soul ties 25

Chapter 3: The Creator's menu 47

Chapter 4: Appointed for the reset 59

Chapter 5: Daily devotionals 79

Chapter 6: Breaking the chain of Babylon 89

Chapter 7: After the reset – how to eat for life 97

Chapter 8: Daily devotionals Pt. 2 105

Chapter 9: Temple prayers for purification 111

Chapter 10: The spiritual science of food 119

Chapter 11: Scriptures for deliverance and healing 129

Chapter 12: The government of healing 137

Bonus 143

About the author 151

Glossary 152

References 154

Addition Research 157

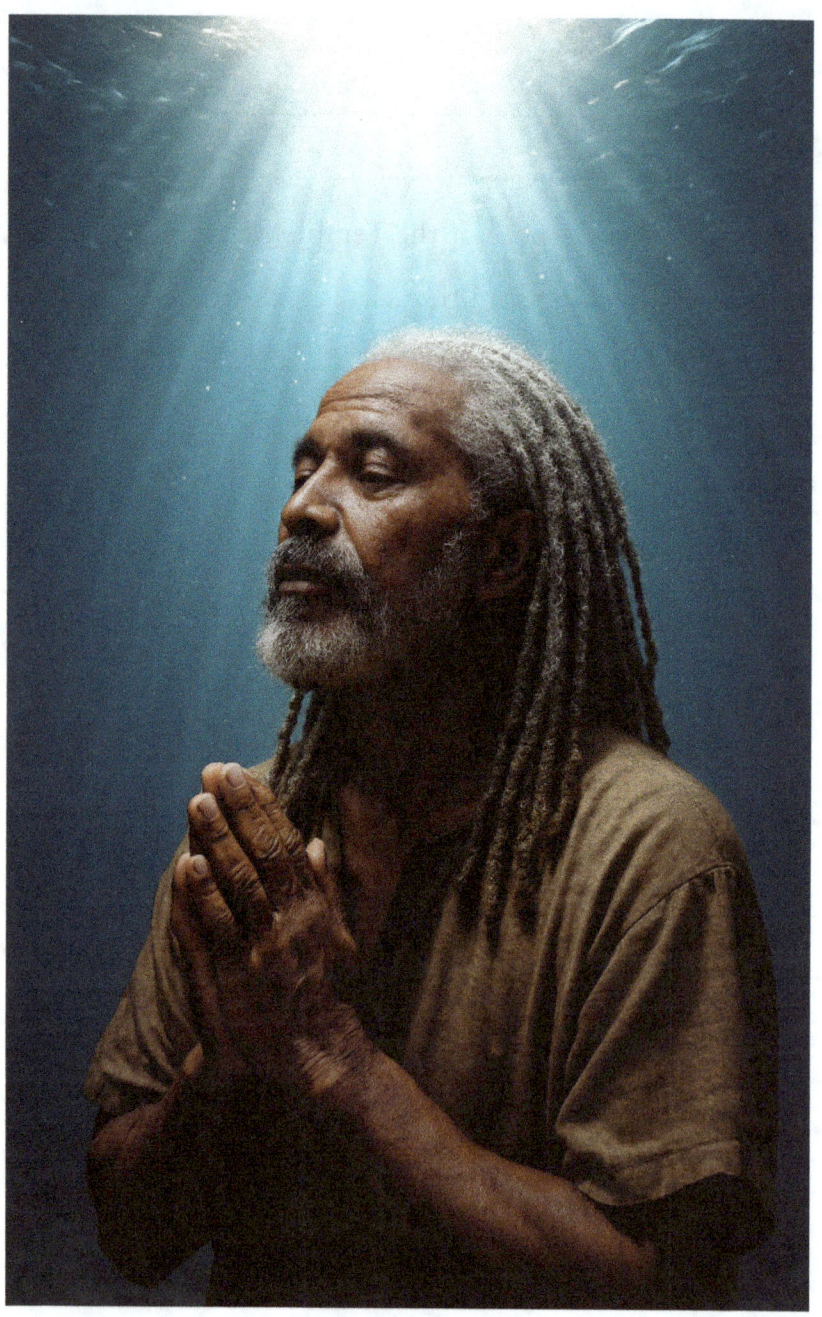

FOREWORD

Many thoughts cross my mind as I think back on the beginning of the 2007 PFA School of Ministry. As the primary instructor, I closely evaluated incoming students. One young man in particular stood out. He was somewhat angry and questioned why he even had to attend. He said his pastor made it mandatory for all of the church's leaders to participate. He argued that he wasn't clergy—he was just the Minister of Music.

As time went by, that young man began to engage enthusiastically in class activities. The anger faded, and by the end of his time with me, he had become my best student. That young man is the author of this book, Pastor Brian Wright, Sr.

Our society has been overwhelmed with an onslaught of addiction. It seems as though we have been ambushed by a multitude of nemeses. There is an ever-increasing incidence of death associated with these addictions, and this epidemic cannot be ignored. Unfortunately, the assault is not subsiding—it's escalating. Addictions take many forms: alcoholism, narcotic drugs, tobacco, over-the-counter medications, and pharmaceutical abuse. There are also sex addicts, thrill-seekers, and those entrapped in perversions and masochism. People are addicted to spending, clothing, automobiles, technology devices—even gambling.

The need for detox, reset, and renewal is real. This is not an imagined situation crying out for a miraculous fix—it's a spiritual and societal emergency.

Pastor Wright has spent a lifetime helping people. In addition to being a minister of the gospel, he is a professional social worker with a Master's degree in Social Work. He is a qualified clinician who actually cares for the people he serves. His empathy for humanity qualifies him to present this important work.

This book is a significant contribution to the healing of both the physical body and the spiritual being. Pastor Wright has worked with a wide range of age groups and demographics. He has served in public schools as well as psychological clinical practices. His willingness to do in-home therapy in addition to hospital-based care contributes to his well-rounded approach in presenting real solutions to a growing crisis.

Pastor Wright's life before salvation also contributes to his authority to speak on detoxification and rehabilitation. His knowledge is not only clinical—it's experiential. His extensive understanding of the steps needed for total rehabilitation is evident in the meticulous manner he lays out this program. His insights on returning to our Creator's original dietary design are both powerful and enlightening. His exposition of spiritual truths echoes the in-depth conversations and dialogues we've shared over the years.

As he discusses reclaiming the Spirit, Pastor Wright deals with the fundamental reason Yeshua came out of eternity and stepped into time—to reconnect our spirit with the Father.

As society grapples with AI, robotics, and other advances in technology, we've drifted farther from natural nutrition and healing. Our dependency on science has led us toward synthetic cures instead of natural remedies. Processed food has become our norm rather than the exception. There is an urgent need to detox, reset, and renew.

This book explains why we must do this, the value of doing it, and how to do it in practical, life-changing ways. I highly recommend this work for all who are serious about living long, living strong, and living in alignment with the One who created us.

Shalom,

Bishop Ronald D. Roston, D.D.

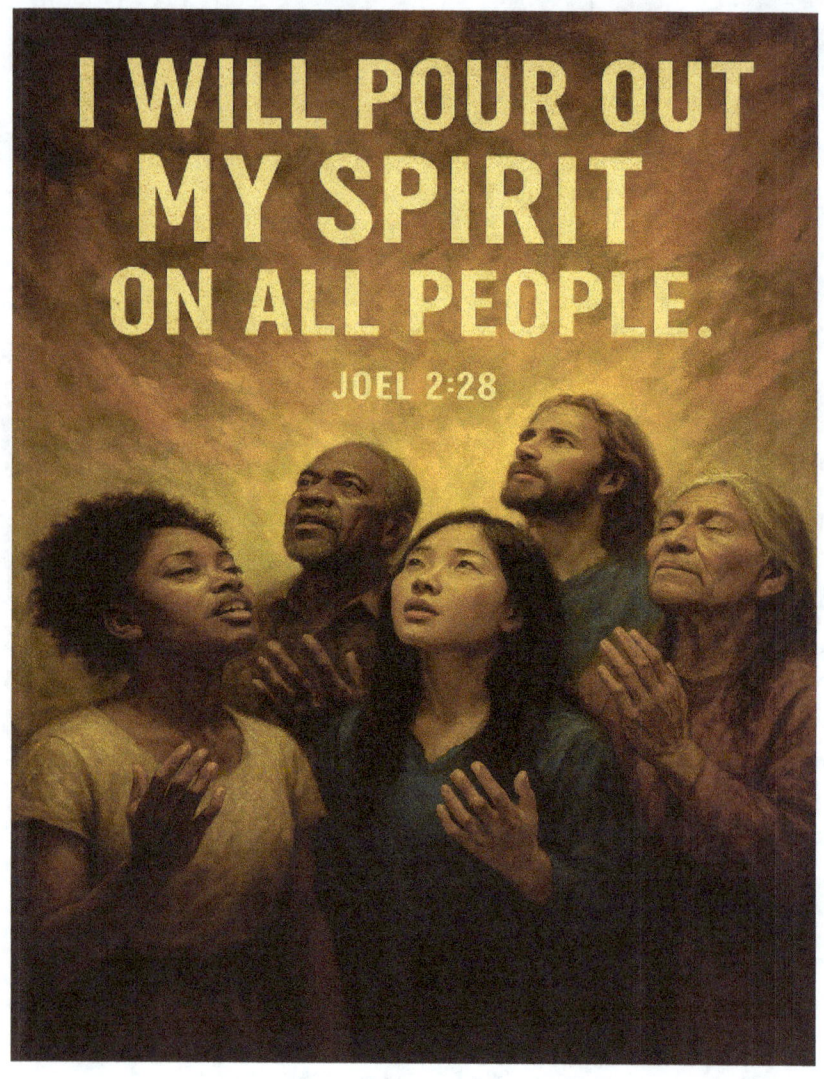

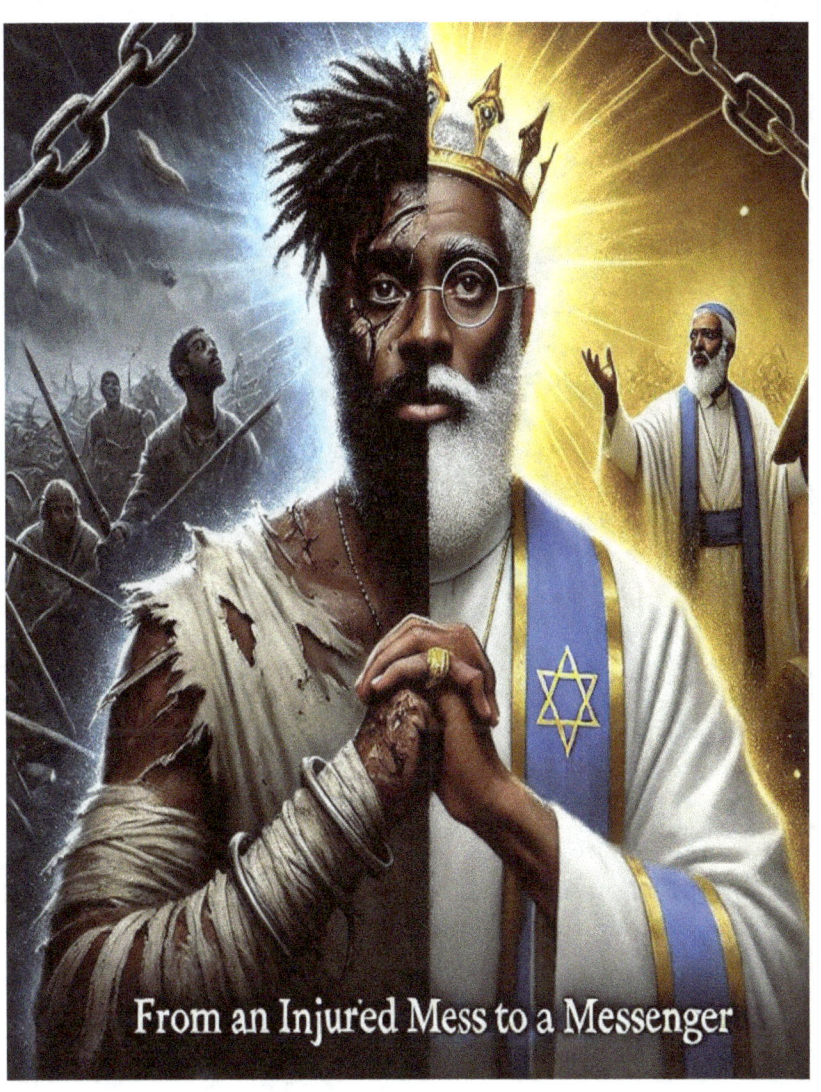

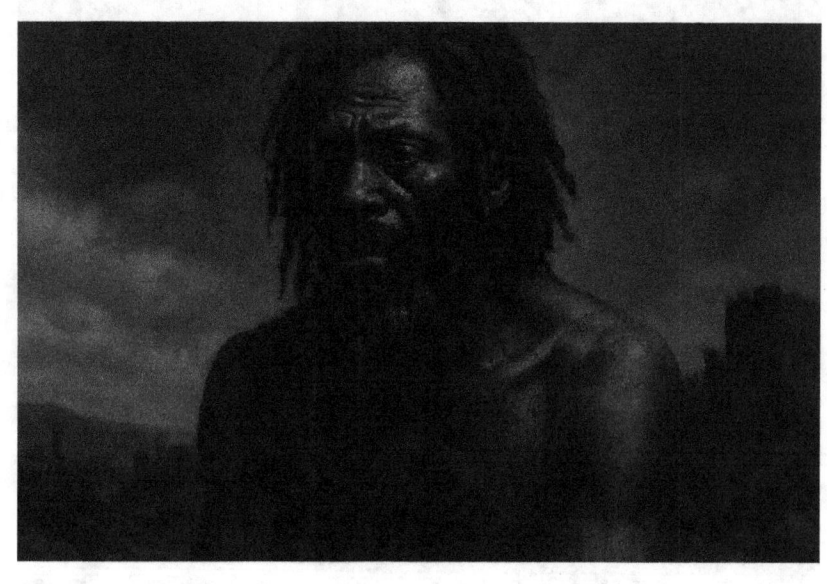

PREFACE

"A Divine Disruption"

I didn't set out to write this book. I was called to it. It started in the quiet. It started in my body. It started when YAH (The LORD) allowed me to be shaken so that I might awaken. This isn't a wellness guide. This isn't just about food. This is a spiritual clarion call for the remnant.

I've seen loss. I've walked through fire. I've survived addiction, buried my sons 19 days apart in February 2013, and faced near-death with nothing but faith and The Ruach Ha'Qodesh (Holy Spirit) whispering, "Your work is not yet done." The Temple Reset was born in the silence between those words. This message is not mine alone. It belongs to every prophet, pastor, parent, and praying believer who knows there is more—more clarity, more peace, more obedience, and more presence.

Babylon has fed us poison; many of us, unknowingly, have eaten it. This is your invitation to unlearn what the world taught you about food, about health, about identity, and return to what YAH (The LORD) always intended. This is a call to prepare your body for the glory He is pouring out. This is about stewardship. This is about sanctification. This is about becoming the kind of dwelling place where the Most High doesn't just visit—He abides. Let this not just be a book you read. Let it be a door you walk through.

Shalom (Peace),

Brian Wright Sr.

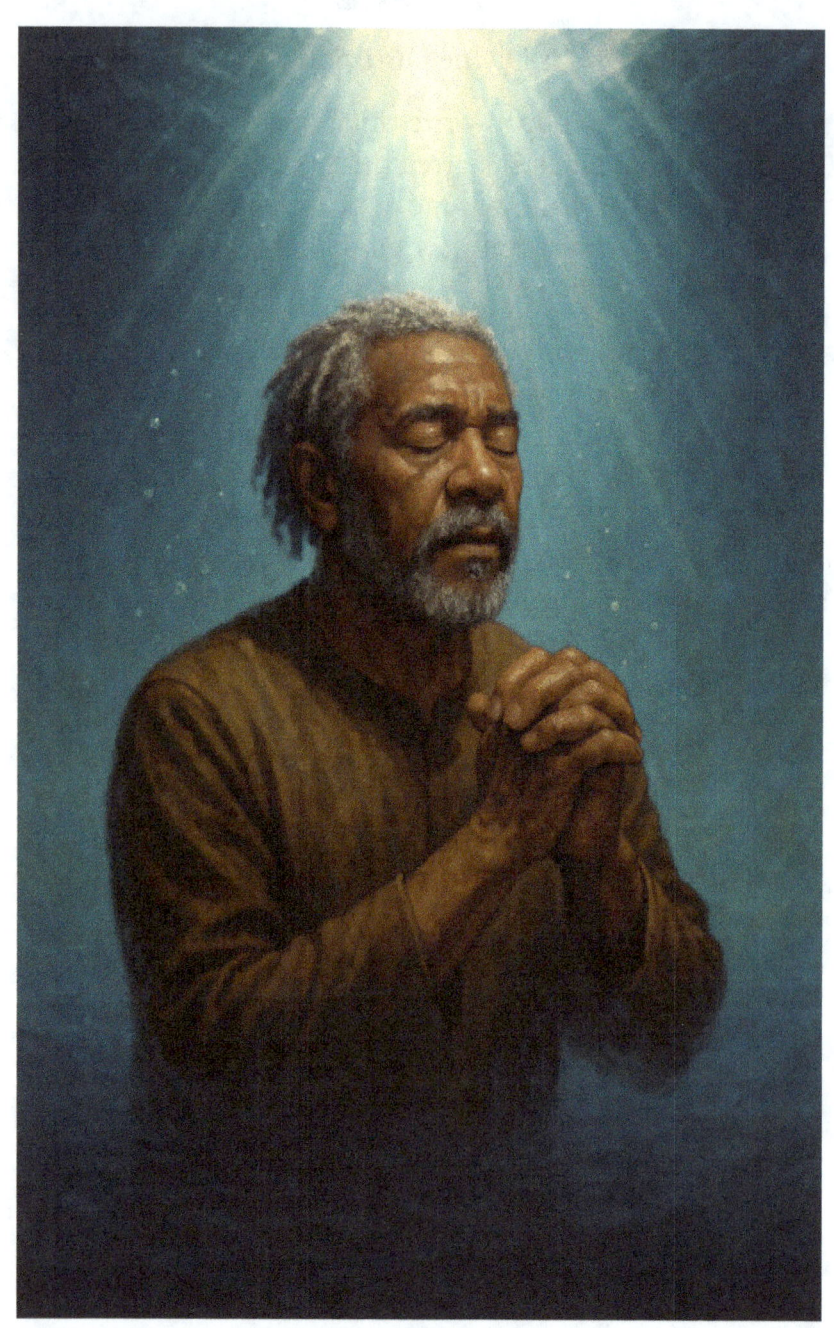

INTRODUCTION

The Temple Reset is a combination of personal experience shared through testimony, research based evidence, scripture from wherever The Ruach Ha'Qodesh (Holy Spirit) has led me, and obedience to Him!

"Before I formed you in the womb I knew you, before you were born I set you apart; I appointed as a prophet to the nations."

— Jeremiah 1:5 (NIV)

I'm partial to The Message Bible as it reads, Before I shaped you in the womb, I knew all about you. Before you saw the light of day I had Holy plans for you: A prophet to the nations. I went to Yah (The LORD) in the process of writing The Temple Reset. He shed light on the fact that in my formal training as a Master Social Worker, my educational process taught me about Human Development / the Life Cycle Model for life. Likewise, there is Spiritual growth and development process. Through my own deliverance, spiritual growth and maturity I have been inspired to write what the Spirit leads me to write. Ruach Ha'Qodesh aka The Holy Spirit led me to Jeremiah and to the understanding of how what was written then relates to us today.

Appointed by Yahuah aka Jehovah

The Word for Yah's (The LORD) people for such a time as now is live a life of purpose on purpose. We must be intentional in this process to reap the fullness of the benefits related to the purpose for The Temple Reset: Detoxing our bodies, Renewing the Mind, Reclaiming the Spirit.

You are who, and what you are by purpose. Yah (The LORD) wants for us to live with focus and discipline, intentionally live for Yah (The LORD). Despite what the world says about who you are know that you are, who Yah (The LORD) says you are. You are who you are not in spite of yourself but because of whose you are.

The wonderful thing about this verse of scripture is that it speaks to Yahuah (God, LORD, or Jehovah), as all-knowing or His omniscience. He already knew Jeremiah's strengths and weaknesses as He also knows ours. He already knew (like Jeremiah) we would possess what He wants to use in these trying perilous times. Just like Jeremiah, there are those of us in whom Yah (The LORD) had set aside a special task which He would give us later in the course of our lives. What this means for us is that though we are not prophets like Jeremiah, we are human beings like him created in Yah's (The LORD) image.

The Word of God in Genesis 1:26 *"Then God said let us make man in our image, in our likeness, and let them rule over the fish of the sea and the birds of the air over the livestock, over all the earth and over all the creatures that move along the ground."* Yah (The LORD) knows each of us, what our strengths, weaknesses, abilities and limitations would be. He knew us even before the foundation of the world.

He has appointed us to become like Yahusha aka Jesus Christ as we follow in the bloodstained footsteps of Yahusha Hamaaschiach (Jesus Christ).

"For those God foreknew He also predestined to become conformed to the image of His Son that he might be among the firstborn among many brothers . And those He predestined, he also called: those he called, he also justified and those he justified he also glorified."

— Romans 8:29-30

There was an appointed day and time for your deliverance or reset. There is also an appointed time for your works. The Ruach Ha'Qodesh (Holy Spirit) is a Gentleman. It is up to us whether or not we accept Yah's (The LORD) appointment just as it was up to Jeremiah.

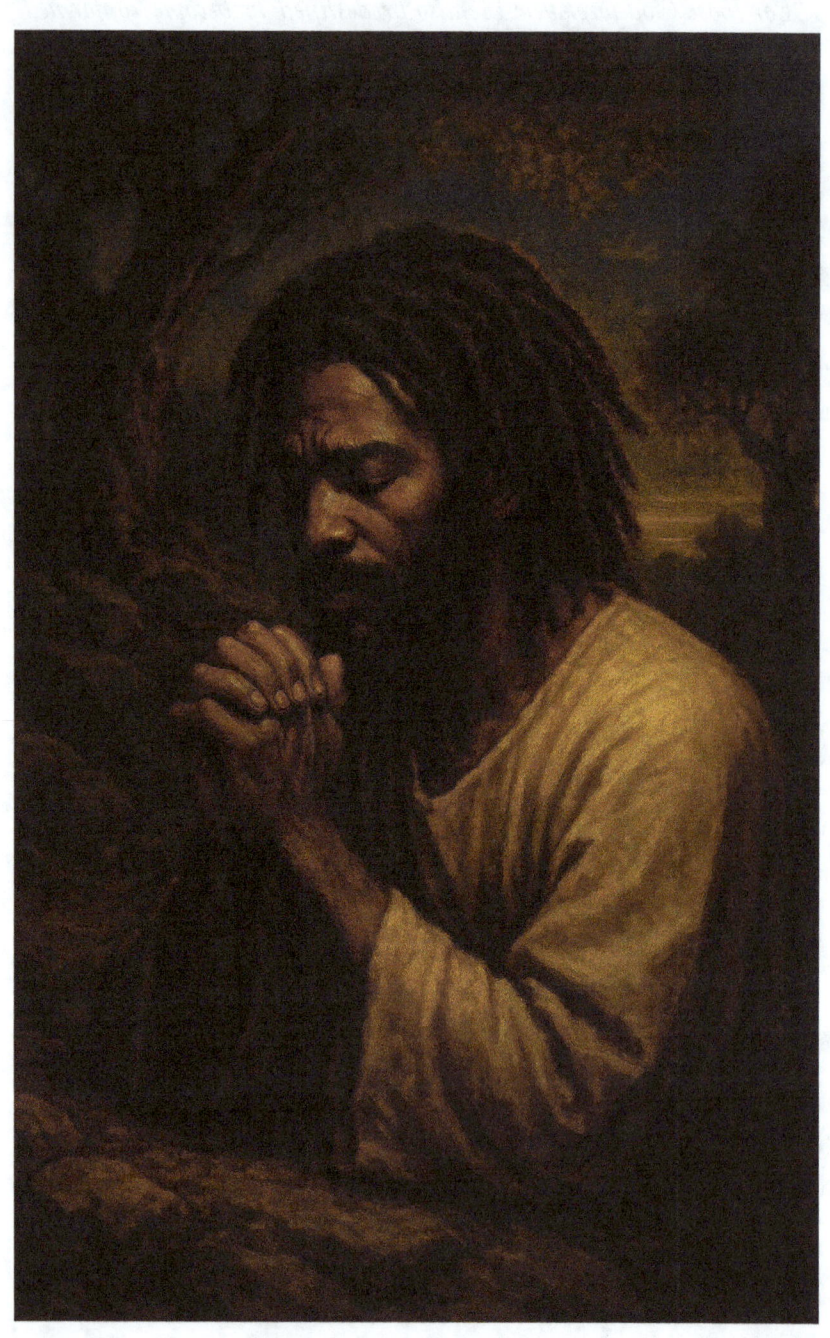

Chapter One

THE PURPOSE OF THE TEMPLE RESET

This is not just a book. This is not just a plan. This is a prophetic assignment. Purpose is the reason or intent of the manufacturer. Yahuah (God, LORD, or Jehovah) is the manufacturer of mankind! Our body is a Temple.

The Temple Reset was born in a moment of divine interruption. It came out of sickness, healing, through dreams, through moments of silence, through fasts I didn't initiate but could no longer avoid. It came through questions and answers I had carried silently for years:

Am I alone in asking "What is wrong with me? Why can't I break through? Why does it feel like I'm stuck in the same patterns—spiritually, physically, emotionally?" The answer came like a whisper and a wind: "Reset the Temple."

THE TEMPLE RESET

What began as a personal conviction became a Kingdom commission. I realized that YAH (The LORD) wasn't just speaking to me—He was speaking through me, to the remnant. To the prophets who had become sluggish. To the intercessors who had grown weary. To the leaders carrying silent pain in overfed, undernourished bodies. To the preachers who have been preaching for hundreds of years information rooted in indoctrination.

To those who knew their calling, like me, but couldn't access the clarity to walk in it fully. This is the reset of body, mind, and spirit. This is the undoing of Babylon's grip and the return to Heaven's blueprint. This is what The Ruach (The Spirit of God) whispered to me in the quiet: "Before I return, I will raise up those who prepare My dwelling place."

You are the dwelling place. The Temple of the Most High! It's high time we, with intentionality, become the practical application of the Word which we preach and teach. Not saying that some don't, but even we can benefit from researching what we were told and not just accept it as, for lack of a better term, the inerrant Gospel!

Too many of us have treated our bodies like rental spaces. We use them. We live in them. We don't truly honor them. We patch holes in the walls with temporary diets, ignore the leaky plumbing of stress and trauma, and expect The Ruach (The Spirit of God) of Yah (The LORD) to dwell in what we ourselves wouldn't move into.

Yah (The LORD) is not looking for temporary residence—He is looking for permanent residence. He will not dwell in a temple we refuse to care for. Ownership says,

CHAPTER ONE - THE PURPOSE OF THE TEMPLE RESET

"This body is not mine; it belongs to the Most High." Occupation says, "I'll do what I want—it's mine."

Ownership leads to stewardship. Occupation leads to self-destruction. "Truth not only informs—it transforms." As my Uncle John used to say to me when I would expound as if I really knew what I was talking about, that which I thought was keen knowledge. He'd say "Life is an ever-learning process!"

This chapter calls us to return to the foundational truth: We are stewards, not owners. Stewards are accountable. This is not about perfection. It's about posture. It's about understanding that the way we treat our body is spiritual. It's worship. It's warfare. It's a witness. This is your reset.

When the Temple Shook

From February 2nd through the 5th, I found myself in the Atlanta VA. A couple of weeks prior, I kept getting up multiple times throughout the night to urinate. I thought it was weird because it was different. Looking back—because hindsight is always 20/20—I now recall a never-ending thirst. I noticed that when I was driving, my vision became increasingly blurred. I felt lethargic. The feeling reminded me of when I was diagnosed with Sarcoidosis back in 2008.

I figured it was a flare-up, but the vision got worse. I didn't feel safe driving, which was how I earned my living at the time, working for Lyft. I called the VA Nurse Line and was instructed to get to the emergency room immediately. I called for an ambulance and was transported to the Atlanta VA.

Upon arrival, I was taken straight to the ICU. I didn't even realize I was in ICU until a nurse told me after being there for a couple of days. The team was focused on lowering my blood glucose level—it was 767. My A1C was 13.9. After about three days, I was moved to a regular room. They continued to monitor my levels and, once steady at around 200, I was discharged.

I know now that was still high—but it was a sight better than 767. They provided compassionate care and explained that I had been in a hyperosmolar hyperglycemic state (HHS). I asked, "What is that?" I was told HHS occurs when blood glucose levels are too high for too long, causing severe dehydration and confusion. Blood sugar levels are usually over 600 mg/dL. If untreated, HHS can lead to coma.

I felt a sense of relief because I was awake and coherent. I wasn't in a coma. I started praising Yahuah (God, LORD, or Jehovah) for that—especially because I had been in that state for about two weeks before calling the nurse line. I wouldn't drive because of the confusion in my mind, trying to figure things out on my own just what was going on with me! Now, there was clarity.

I reached out to prayer warriors. I even posted on Facebook asking for prayer. The last thing I wanted was to be sick, in a coma, or worse—dead. I kept thinking about my daughter Carmen and other family members, and how my death might impact them. In Carmen's case, I thought, "No! YAH (The LORD)! She's already lost both of her brothers."

As I lay in that hospital bed, I talked to and listened for

CHAPTER ONE - THE PURPOSE OF THE TEMPLE RESET

Ruach Ha'Qodesh (Holy Spirit). I told Him about my deep concern for Carmen. Back in September 2012, I lost my brother Warren to cancer. One hundred and nine days later, my oldest son Maurice Antaughn Bruce was murdered. Nineteen days after burying him, my youngest and only other son, Brian Wright Jr., was also murdered.

These remain unsolved cases by the Pittsburgh, PA Homicide Division. The murders have had a major impact on my family—especially Carmen. She lost both of her brothers. So yes, my concern for her was great. Yah (The LORD) forbid I died! I guess He did because I'm still here on this side of glory. Telling you this part of my story.

I want to emphasize that what I experienced was not just a medical emergency—it was a divine interruption. A reset. My body was crying out for alignment, but so was my spirit. In the stillness of that hospital room, I felt the presence of The Ruach Ha'Qodesh (Holy Spirit) like never before. He reminded me that this was bigger than me; that my story would be used to shake others awake. Even in the ICU, I was being commissioned. Not only to heal—but to help others heal.

So, if you're reading this and you've ever ignored the signs... If you've ever felt the fog, the fatigue, the spiritual silence—know that YAH (The LORD) speaks even in crises. Yes, especially in crises. He's still saying: Reset the Temple.

The Assignment: Why YAH (The LORD) is calling His remnant to detox now? This assignment isn't just personal—it's prophetic. It's not about a health trend. It's about a holy call. The Most High is sounding the alarm to His remnant. He is calling a people out of spiritual sleep, dietary bondage, and cultural compromise.

We have eaten what Babylon served us—physically and spiritually—for too long. We've consumed processed food and processed doctrine. We've settled for **convenience over covenant**. We've forgotten that what we ingest affects how we hear.

Our bodies, our minds, and our spirits have been dulled by the very systems YAH (The LORD) told us to come out from. Now, He is calling us back. Back to Eden. Back to intention. Back to discipline. Back to the sacred understanding that the body is not a tool for indulgence—it is a vessel for glory.

This detox is not just about what we **remove**—it's about what we **restore**! Clarity. Sensitivity to The Ruach (The Spirit of God). Authority. Peace. Healing. Power. Worship.

This is why YAH (The LORD) is calling His remnant to detox now: we must be spiritually sharp for what's ahead. He wants to dwell in a clean temple. There is a harvest to reach and a battle to win. Revival doesn't start in the church—it starts in the temple. The reset begins here. The call is now. The remnant is rising. Selah.

CHAPTER ONE - THE PURPOSE OF THE TEMPLE RESET

THE TEMPLE RESET

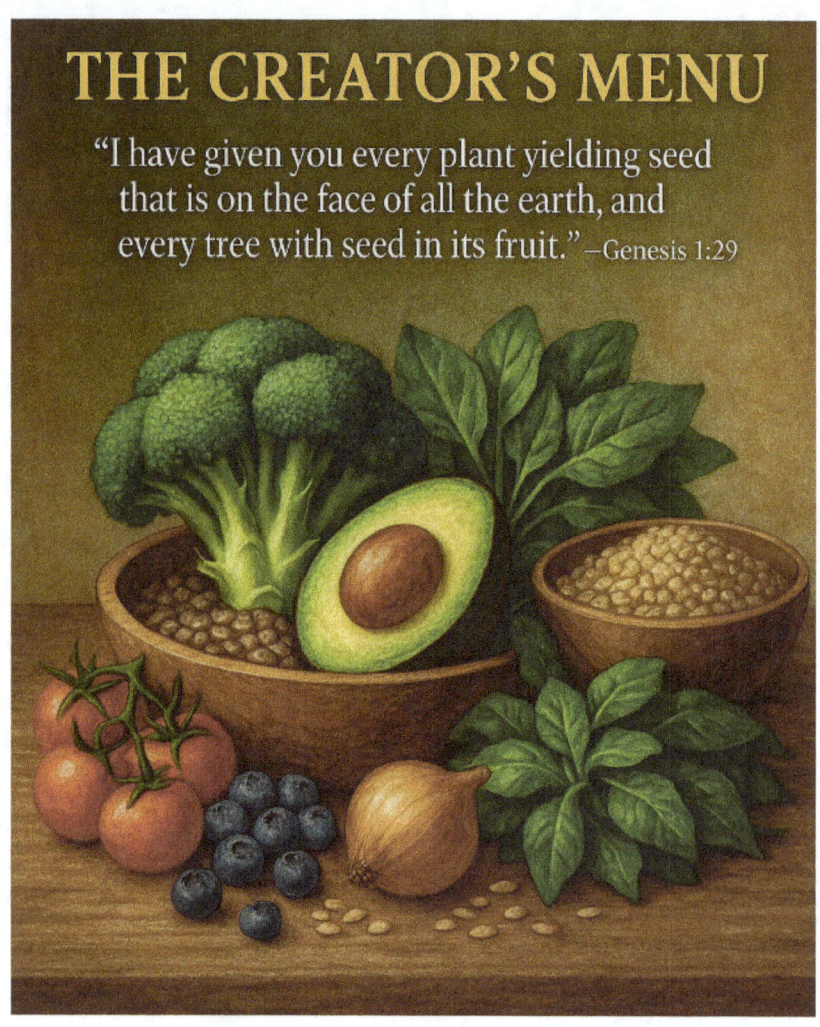

Chapter Two

BREAKING THE SOUL TIES WITH BABYLON'S FOOD SYSTEM

Upon returning home, I began to follow the VA doctors' orders. I was sticking myself daily, checking my BGLs, and taking my insulin shots. Then The Ruach Ha'Qodesh (Holy Spirit) deposited a name in my spirit: *Kimberly Nicole Jackson-Morris*, one of my oldest friends from high school. I remembered how she gave life-giving information when a family member had cancer. That information prolonged her life.

I immediately called her, and she shared something that would become a catalyst for this next phase of the reset. She sent me an assignment via text message: "Research Red 40, Yellow 5, Blue 1, and Aspartame."

I thought, "What? I'm not doing that!" But I obeyed. What I found changed everything.

The Unholy Infiltration: What We've Consumed Without Question

We trusted what was on the shelves. We accepted what was passed down. In doing so, we made agreements with Babylon's food system—unknowingly yoking our temples to chemicals that suppress our clarity, silence our discernment, and invite disease.

These dyes and artificial sweeteners aren't just about taste—they are spiritual tools of distraction and destruction. As the body of Hamaschiach (The Anointed One)— the Anointed One, we've fasted from sin but feasted on poison. We've prayed for healing while consuming what makes us sick. However, YAH (The LORD) is shining a light on the deception.

Below is a breakdown of what I discovered. May it stir your awareness, not fear. May it ignite your obedience to detox. Upon returning home, I began to follow the VA doctor's orders. I was pricking myself daily, checking my BGL's (blood glucose levels), and taking my insulin shots.

I completed her assignment and the results I found are as follows. The side effects of Red 40, Yellow 5, Blue 1, and Aspartame have been widely studied, though opinions on their safety vary. Below is a breakdown of each:

1. Red 40 (Allura Red AC), a common food dye. It is found in a wide variety of processed foods, including

CHAPTER TWO — BREAKING SOUL TIES

candies, soft drinks, cereals, snack foods, dairy products, and even some medications and cosmetics.

Common Side Effects:

- Hyperactivity in children (linked to ADHD, Attention Defict Hyperactivity Disorder symptoms)
- Allergic reactions (hives, skin rash)
- Headaches
- Stomach discomfort

Concerns: Some studies suggest it may cause DNA damage or cancer in high doses, though the FDA (Food and Drug Administration) considers it safe in regulated amounts. The synthetic food dye, Red 40, causes DNA damage, causes colonic inflammation, and impacts the microbiome in mice.

Here's a more detailed list of foods and products that may contain Red Dye 40:

Foods:

- Cereals: Froot Loops, Lucky Charms, Trix, Fruity Pebbles
- Candy and Gum: Skittles, M&Ms, Jolly Rancher, Starburst, Bubblicious
- Snack Foods: Doritos, Flamin' Hot Cheetos, Planters Cheez Balls, Combos Pizzeria Pretzels

- Dairy Products: Flavored milk and yogurts, ice cream, popsicles
- Puddings and Gelatines
- Baked Goods: Cakes, pastries, frosting
- Beverages: Sodas, sports drinks, energy drinks
- Fruit Snacks and Juices
- Condiments and Sauces
- Protein Powders

Other Products

- Over-the-counter medications and vitamins

Cosmetics: Lipstick, eyeliner, eyeshadow, blush, bubble baths, and some kids' toothpastes

- Tattoo inks
- Maraschino cherries
- Jello
- Chewing gum
- Protein powders
- Meat and poultry
- Gelatin

2. Yellow 5 (Tartrazine)Yellow 5 is an artificial food dye added to processed pastries, brightly colored soda, and colored candy. Consuming more than the recommend-

ed amount may cause hyperactivity in children and other health effects over time.

Common Side Effects:

- Hyperactivity in children
- Allergic reactions (hives, asthma symptoms)
- Headaches
- Anxiety or mood changes

Concerns: It has been linked to exacerbating asthma and causing behavioral changes in sensitive individuals.

Yellow 5, also known as tartrazine, is a common food dye found in a wide variety of foods, including candies, sodas, breakfast cereals, and processed snacks, as well as some medications and cosmetics.

Here's a more detailed list of foods and products where you might encounter Yellow 5:

Common Sources:

- Candies and Confections: Brightly colored candies, gummy bears, marshmallows, cotton candy, and hard candies.
- Sodas and Beverages: Flavored sodas, flavored drink mixes, Kool-Aid, Mountain Dew, Gatorade, and Powerade.
- Breakfast Cereals: Sugary breakfast cereals like Cap'n

Crunch and Lucky Charms.

- Snack Foods: Chips, flavored chips (Doritos, Ruffles, Fritos), and other processed snacks.
- Baked Goods and Desserts: Cake mixes, pastries, instant puddings, gelatin desserts, and ice cream.
- Other Foods: Sauces, condiments, pickles, relishes, processed cheeses, and some yogurts.
- Medications: Some pills, syrups and other pharmaceuticals.
- Cosmetics and Personal Care Items

Examples of Brand Names:

- Doritos: (certain flavors)
- Froot Loops
- Lemon-flavored Jello
- Knorr chicken bouillon
- M&Ms
- Starburst
- Mountain Dew
- Gatorade
- Cap'N Crunch
- Lucky Charms
- Sunny D
- Kool-Aid Jammers

- Twinkies

It can be found in a variety of foods, including:

- Cereal
- Sodas
- Gelatines
- Frosting
- Spices
- Sauces
- Yogurt
- Juices

3. Blue 1 (Brilliant Blue FCF) Blue 1, also known as Brilliant Blue FCF, is a synthetic food dye often found in candies, beverages, baked goods, and other processed foods like canned peas and ice cream.

Common Side Effects:

- Allergic reactions (though rare)
- Skin rashes
- Gastrointestinal issues

Concerns: Animal studies have shown potential links to cancer, but no conclusive evidence has been found in humans.

Common Foods and Beverages:

- Candies: Nerds, Skittles, M&Ms, Sour Patch Kids, gummy bears, and other colorful candies
- Beverages: Soft drinks (like Fanta Berry), sports drinks (Gatorade Cool Blue), and flavored juices
- Baked Goods: Pastries, cakes, and cookies
- Canned Goods: Canned peas
- Other Processed Foods: Cereals (like Lucky Charms), ice cream, yogurt, and icings
- Liqueurs: Blue Curaçao
- Snacks: Chips, popcorn, and other processed snacks
- Medications: Some children's medications and even certain prescription drugs may contain FD&C Blue #1
- Other: Salad dressing, condiments, and even some types of smoked salmon

4. Aspartame (Artificial Sweetener) Aspartame, an artificial sweetener, is commonly found in diet sodas, sugar-free gums, powdered drink mixes, and some low-sugar desserts, yogurts, and cereals.

Common Side Effects:

- Headaches
- Dizziness

- Mood changes
- Digestive issues

Concerns:

Long-term studies suggest possible links to cancer, though regulatory bodies like the FDA (Food and Drug Administration) and WHO (World Health Organization) deem it safe in moderate amounts. Individuals with phenylketonuria (PKU) must avoid aspartame entirely, as it contains phenylalanine.

Here's a more detailed list of foods and drinks that may contain Aspartame:

Beverages:

- Diet sodas (e.g., Diet Coke, Coke Zero, Pepsi Max)
- Low-sugar juices
- Flavored sparkling water
- Powdered drink mixes (e.g., Crystal Light)
- Low-calorie coffee sweeteners

Foods:

- Sugar-free chewing gum (e.g., Trident)
- Sugar-free gelatin (e.g., Sugar-free Jell-O)
- Low-sugar desserts
- Reduced-sugar condiments (e.g., Log Cabin Sugar Free Syrup)

- Sugar-free jams
- Flavored yogurts
- Breakfast cereals
- Granola bars
- Low-fat yogurt
- Low-fat flavored milk
- Nutrition bars
- Low-fat or light ice cream and popsicles
- Some prescription and over-the-counter medicines, including chewable vitamins

Final Thoughts:

    These additives are FDA-approved in regulated amounts but can have adverse effects, especially in sensitive individuals. The EU (European Union) requires warning labels on products with certain artificial dyes, especially for children. In contrast to the EU, the U.S. FDA had a different approach, previously stating dyes were safe. However, as of early 2025, the FDA has banned Red No. 3 in U.S. food products and is working to phase out other dyes by 2026 based on similar concerns, though compliance is voluntary. It's wise to limit consumption of artificial colors and sweeteners, opting for natural alternatives when possible. The following is a list of natural alternatives to these ingredients?

    Natural alternatives to Red 40, Yellow 5, Blue 1, and Aspartame that are healthier and can often provide even better flavor and color without the harmful side effects.

Natural Alternatives for Artificial Food Dyes:

Red 40
- Beet Juice Powder
- Beets
- Pomegranate Juice
- Pomegranate
- Hibiscus Extract
- Hibiscus Flower

Yellow 5
- Turmeric Powder
- Turmeric
- Saffron
- Saffron Flower
- Annatto
- Seeds from the Achiote Tree

Blue 1
- Spirulina
- Blue-Green Algae
- Butterfly Pea Flower

- Dried Butterfly Pea Flowers
- Purple Sweet Potato Juice
- Sweet Potatoes

Natural Sweetener Alternatives for Aspartame:
Artificial Sweetener Natural Alternative Benefits
- Stevia

    Zero calories, plant-based, no blood sugar spike:
- Monk Fruit

    Zero calories, antioxidant-rich
- Raw Honey

    Natural energy booster, antimicrobial
- Maple Syrup

    Full of minerals, antioxidants
- Dates

    Natural sweetness, fiber-rich

If you're looking for natural flavor enhancers, try:
- Vanilla Bean
- Cinnamon
- Mint
- Lemon or Orange Zest

CHAPTER TWO — BREAKING SOUL TIES

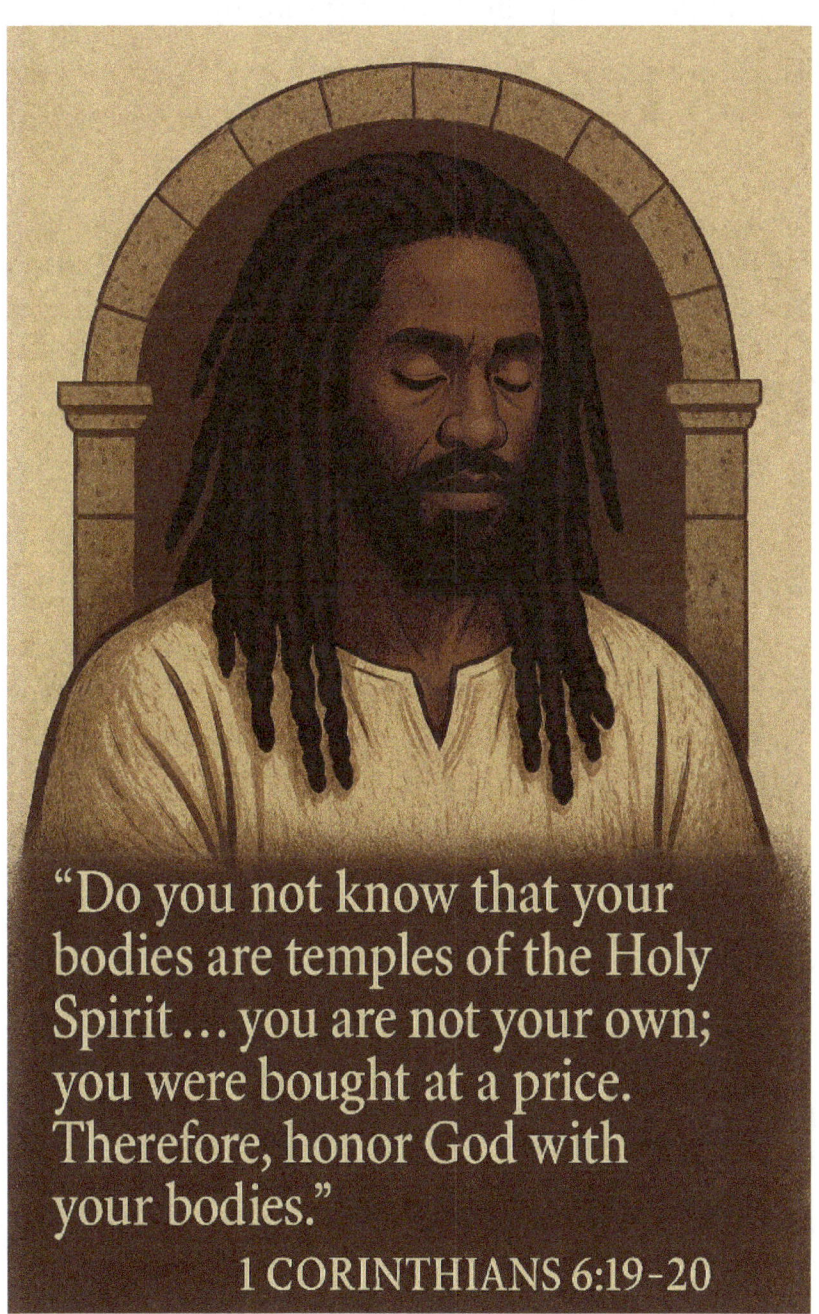

"Do you not know that your bodies are temples of the Holy Spirit… you are not your own; you were bought at a price. Therefore, honor God with your bodies."

1 CORINTHIANS 6:19-20

Why This Matters Spiritually

The Word says in 1 Corinthians 6:19-20: *"Do you not know that your bodies are temples of the Holy Spirit?"*

What we put into our bodies affects not only our health but our ability to hear from the Most High. Returning to the natural provisions of Yah's (The LORD) creation brings us back into alignment with His divine design. "Temple Cleanse" Shopping List with natural foods, herbs, and drinks to detox from these chemicals.

Temple Cleanse Shopping List

"For the temple of God is holy, which temple ye are."

— 1 Corinthians 3:17

This Temple Cleanse is designed to help detox your body from artificial chemicals like Red 40, Yellow 5, Blue 1, Aspartame, and other toxins—while restoring your body with what the Most High originally intended.

Revelation Moment

The devil's agenda has always been to corrupt what God created—even down to what we eat and drink. These man-made chemicals are not just harming our bodies, they're blocking our ability to fully connect with YAH (The LORD).

When you detox from Babylon's food system and return to The Creator's Menu, your spiritual ears will open like never before.

CHAPTER TWO — BREAKING SOUL TIES

The Temple Reset: 7-Day Detox + Scripture Devotional

"Beloved, I wish above all things that thou mayest prosper and be in health, even as thy soul prospereth."

— 3 John 1:2

From Agreement to Alignment

Why This Matters Spiritually

1 Corinthians 6:19-20 reminds us: *"Do you not know that your bodies are temples of the Holy Spirit... you are not your own; you were bought at a price. Therefore, honor God with your bodies."*

What you put in your body is not a neutral act—it's worship or rebellion. Babylon doesn't care about your temple, but the Most High does, and is calling us to rise from this dietary captivity into alignment with His original design.

This isn't just about "eating clean." This is about walking in Kingdom clarity. Returning to Eden's provision. Restoring the frequency of your temple to hear from YAH (The LORD) again.

Temple Cleanse Tools:

What the Most High Has Already Provided

1. Cleanse the Blood (Detox System)
- Beets (Fresh or Powder)
- Dandelion Root Tea
- Burdock Root

THE TEMPLE RESET

- Chlorophyll Drops
- Lemon + Ginger Water
- Spirulina Powder

2. Cleanse the Gut (Remove Artificial Sweeteners & Dyes)

- Sea Moss Gel
- Flaxseed
- Psyllium Husk Powder
- Apple Cider Vinegar (with the Mother)
- Organic Dates (Natural Sweetener)
- Raw Honey
- Coconut Sugar
- Herbal Laxative Tea (Senna + Peppermint)

3. Rebuild the Temple (Nourish & Restore)

- Organic Fruits (Blueberries, Pineapple, Apples, Grapes)
- Leafy Greens (Kale, Spinach, Arugula)
- Avocados (Healthy Fats)
- Almonds & Walnuts
- Raw Pumpkin Seeds
- Quinoa
- Chickpeas (for Protein)

4. Hydrate the Temple (Living Water)

CHAPTER TWO — BREAKING SOUL TIES

- Spring Water (pH 7.4 or Higher)
- Coconut Water
- Lemon + Mint Infused Water
- Hibiscus Tea
- Ginger Tea
- Cucumber Water

5. Renew the Mind (Mental & Spiritual Detox)

- Moringa Powder (Brain Food)
- Ashwagandha (Stress Relief)
- Holy Basil Tea

Daily Meditation on Psalm 51:10

"Create in me a clean heart, O God, and renew a right spirit within me."

7-Day Temple Cleanse Daily Plan Time
What to Consume

Upon Waking

- Lemon + Ginger Water (Detox)

Morning

- Sea Moss + Spirulina Smoothie

Midday

- Burdock Root or Dandelion Tea

Afternoon

THE TEMPLE RESET

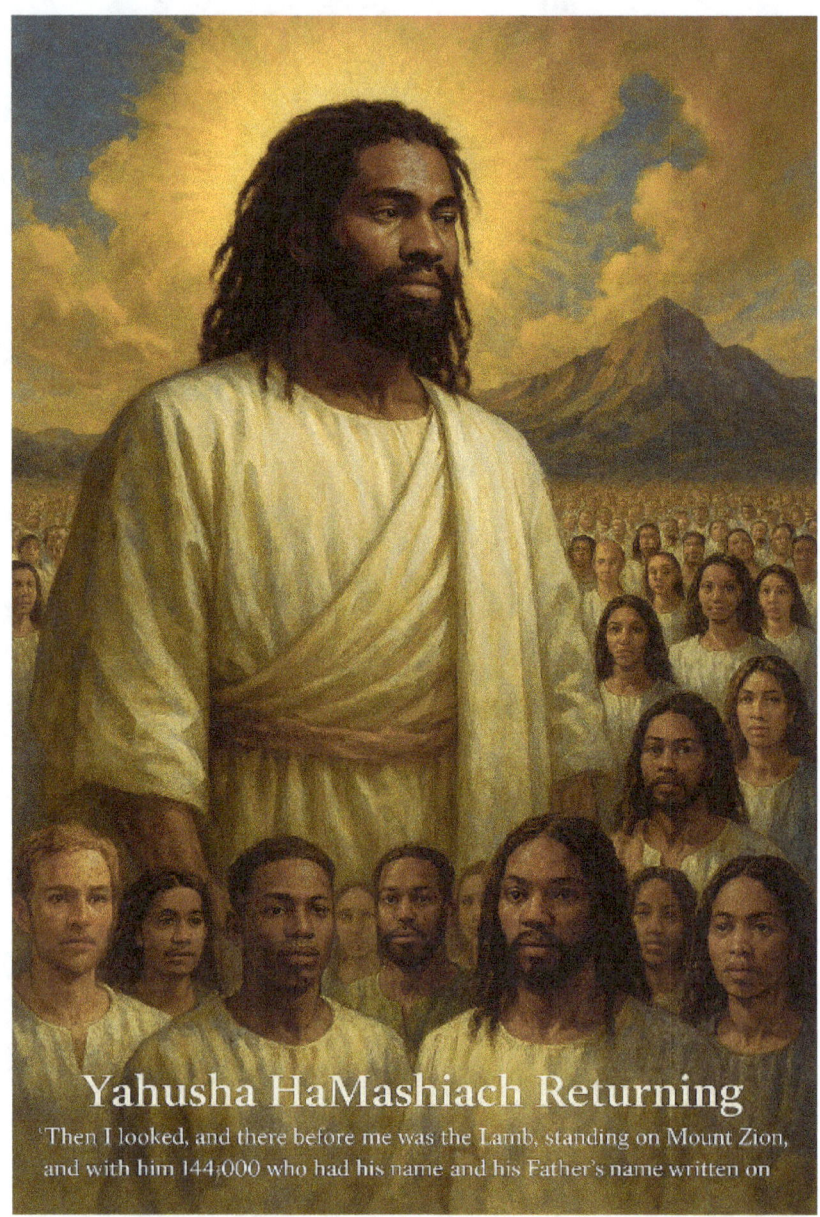

Yahusha HaMashiach Returning

'Then I looked, and there before me was the Lamb, standing on Mount Zion, and with him 144,000 who had his name and his Father's name written on

CHAPTER TWO — BREAKING SOUL TIES

THE BABYLONIAN DETOX

A PROPHETIC CALL TO HUNGER

Prophetic Insight:

Many of the chronic issues in the body of believers today—foggy thinking, spiritual dullness, lack of stamina in prayer—are not just spiritual attacks. They are dietary agreements with Babylon. The Reset begins when we repent... not just in prayer, but at the plate.

Return to the menu of Heaven. The garden is still calling. The Tree of Life is still avaiable. And the Father's desire is that we taste and see that He is good— even in what we eat.

John 7:38

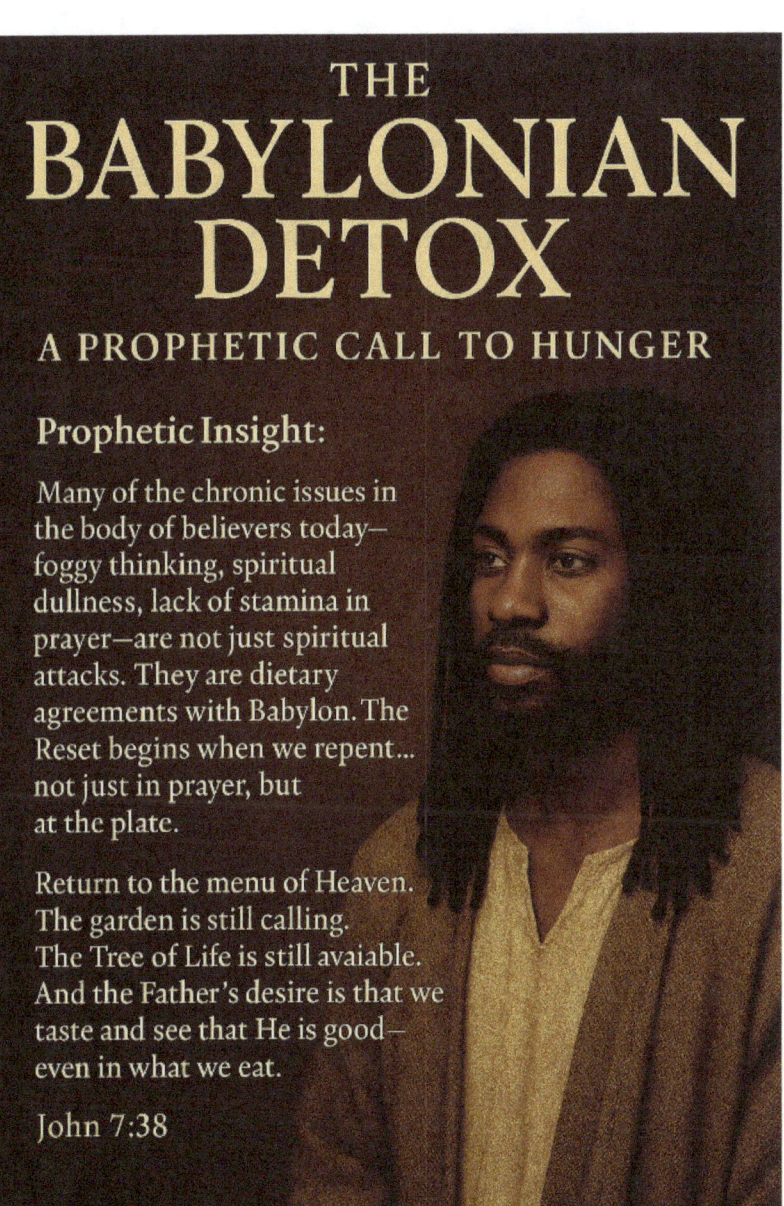

THE TEMPLE RESET

- Fresh Salad + Quinoa + Avocado

Evening

- Detox Tea + Fruit

Before Bed

- Psalm 51 Meditation + Coconut Water

Bonus: Prayers for the Temple

Morning: "Father, purify this temple for Your glory."

Evening: "Create in me a clean heart and renew a right spirit within me."

What This Cleanse Will Do:

Flush out artificial toxins

- Clear brain fog
- Improve energy & sleep
- Restore spiritual clarity

Align the temple with Heaven's frequency. These are not just ingredients. They are intercessors in your bloodstream. They are repairers of the breach. They are Heaven's original medicine—hidden in plain sight, waiting for the remnant to rediscover.

Revelation Moment: A Prophetic Call to Detox

The devil's tactic has always been to pervert what

CHAPTER TWO — BREAKING SOUL TIES

God creates. He entered the garden with a question, *"Did God really say?"* He continues today with additives, dyes, and lies. We are not ignorant of his devices. The Ruach (The Spirit of God) is exposing them, and the "Temple Reset" is your invitation to realign. You were not created to live in fog, fatigue, inflammation, and confusion. You were created to walk in clarity, strength, and sacred awareness. This is your wake-up call. This is your soul tiebreaker. This is your reset.

Bonus Revelation

The Temple Reset is directly tied to what YAH (The LORD) is doing in this hour: He's calling His remnant to purify the temple before the return of Yahusha Hamaschiach (Jesus Christ).

The very same chemicals you're detoxing from are the ones the Pharmaceutical Industry and Food Industry use to weaken the body and keep the mind in bondage.

This is not just about what's on your plate—this is about breaking strongholds over your purpose, your perception, and your power.

"Beloved, I wish above all things that thou mayest prosper and be in health, even as thy soul prospereth."

—3 John 1:2

THE TEMPLE RESET

Chapter Three

THE CREATOR'S MENU

"Then God said, 'Behold, I have given you every herb bearing seed, which is on the face of all the earth, and every tree whose fruit yields seed; to you it shall be for food.'"

—Genesis 1:29"

YAH (The LORD) never intended for us to live off chemicals, dyes, and preservatives. From the beginning, He gave us a menu—not made by man, but crafted by the Creator. It was a divine blueprint for nourishment, healing, and spiritual clarity.

In Eden, there was no processed food, no additives, no artificial sweeteners. There was fruit. There were herbs. There were seeds. All of them carried life.

The Creator's Menu was designed to:

- Sustain the body
- Sharpen the mind
- Align the spirit

When mankind drifted from the garden, we drifted from the menu. We began to eat what was profitable for corporations but poisonous for our temples. We chose convenience over covenant, cravings over calling.

Returning to the Creator's Menu is not a diet. It's a decision—to trust YAH's (The LORD) original design more than the world's processed replacements.

This chapter is a call to: (A) Rediscover the foods YAH (The LORD) called "good." (B) Learn how certain fruits, herbs, and grains affect your spiritual and physical health. (C) Realign your taste buds with Heaven's table

Let the garden speak again. Let Eden rise within your temple. Let the Creator's Menu become your lifestyle. This isn't just about what to eat. It's about how to live. Let's open the scroll of Genesis 1:29, and eat what was written.

The Garden Still Speaks: Eating with Intention

When we return to Genesis 1:29, we aren't just revisiting ancient history—we are reclaiming a sacred rhythm. YAH (The LORD) gave us every seed-bearing plant and fruit-bearing tree as food, not just for survival, but for thriving.

CHAPTER THREE - THE CREATOR'S MENU

The colors, textures, and flavors in Eden were not just about pleasure. They were about purpose. Blueberries for the brain. Pomegranates for the blood. Garlic to purify. Honey to energize. Olive oil to anoint.

What Babylon calls "organic," Heaven calls original. What the world labels as a diet, Heaven defines as dominion.

To return to the Creator's Menu is to:

- See food as fuel for prophecy
- Recognize plants as prayer partners
- Treat each bite as an act of worship

Foods of the Covenant Here are a few examples of how specific foods from the Creator's Menu restore the body and align the spirit:

» **Leafy Greens (Spinach, Kale, Arugula)** - Detoxify the blood and support clarity in prayer.

» **Grapes** - Symbol of covenant, full of antioxidants, aid digestion and reduce inflammation.

» **Nuts & Seeds (Chia, Flax, Pumpkin)** - Contain omega-3s that support brain health and hormonal balance.

» **Herbs (Basil, Cilantro, Parsley)** - Remove heavy metals, aid liver cleansing, refresh the breath of life.

» **Root Vegetables (Beets, Carrots, Sweet Potatoes)** - Ground the body, stabilize blood sugar, bring endurance

Every food from the Creator carries intention. When we bless what He intended, we align our health with His holiness. The Creator's Menu: Returning to Heaven's Table

> *"And God said, Behold, I have given you every herb bearing seed... to you it shall be for food."*
>
> — *Genesis 1:29*

- Before there was a temple, there was a table.
- Before there was a priest, there was a garden.
- Before the Law, there was provision.

Genesis 1:29 is more than a menu—it's a mandate.

It is Heaven's original prescription for health, healing, and holiness. It's time we return to the table YAH (The LORD) prepared. Point 1: YAH's (The LORD) Provision Was Always Pure

"Behold, I have given you..." YAH (The LORD) didn't suggest food—He gave it. Provision is part of His nature. What He gave wasn't polluted, preserved, or processed. It was pure.

When you receive food with reverence, you return to the rhythm of the garden. Application: Stop calling Babylon's food "normal." Go back to what's natural. The Seed Is Sacred "Every herb bearing seed..." Seeds are sacred—they carry life in dormant form. What YAH (The LORD) gives us in seed form, Babylon tries to manufacture in a lab.

CHAPTER THREE - THE CREATOR'S MENU

GMO culture wants to clone, patent, and sell what YAH (The LORD) already gave freely. GMO (Genetically Modified Organisms, are organisms with genetic material (DNA) changed through genetic engineering, often involving DNA transfer from one organism to another. What comes from a seed carries a spiritual blueprint of original design. Food Was Always Meant to Be Functional "To you it shall be for food." Not for addiction. Not for emotional escape. Not for bondage. Food is meant to fuel the body, free the mind, and align the spirit. Not the additives that put our health at risk! The reset begins when we let Eden be our model again. What's feeding you—the garden or the system?

Closing Declaration:

"Father, I return to Your table. I reject the substitutes of this world. Let the food I eat be a form of worship—and let my body become the altar. I receive Your menu. I realign with Your design. In Yahusha's (Jesus) name, Amein (Amen)."

Prophetic Insight: Many of the chronic issues in the body of believers today—foggy thinking, spiritual dullness, lack of stamina in prayer—are not just spiritual attacks. They are dietary agreements with Babylon. We have unknowingly signed contracts with counterfeit nourishment, trusting processed goods over the provisions of YAH (The LORD). These agreements weaken our spiritual sensitivity, dull our discernment, and shorten the duration of our consecration.

The Temple Reset begins when we repent, not just in prayer, but at the plate. Because every bite is a yes or no to alignment. We can't fast for clarity and then feast on confusion. We can't ask for deliverance while ingesting what keeps us bound. This is why the adversary infiltrates the food system—because he knows a polluted temple produces a muted voice.

When you detox from Babylon's table and return to the Creator's Menu, your prayers sharpen, your dreams return, and your mind clears. You begin to hunger for righteousness—not just in spirit, but in substance.

Return to the menu of Heaven. The garden is still calling. The Tree of Life is still available. It is the Father's desire is that we taste and see that He is good—even in what we eat.

Let he that has an ear hear what Yah (The LORD) is saying! *"Whether therefore ye eat, or drink, or whatsoever ye do, do all to the glory of God."* —1 Corinthians 10:31. Oh boy! Here comes the preacher! Introduction: The Apostle Paul isn't just giving diet advice, he's revealing a Kingdom principle.

In everything we do, even in the mundane, there is a divine opportunity for worship. So, what if our eating and drinking isn't neutral, rather spiritual?

That includes what's on your plate and what's in your cup. Eating and drinking are not neutral—they are spiritual. Every plate is an altar. Every cup is a covenant reminder. Worship doesn't begin at the sanctuary; it begins at the table.

Food is never "just food." In the Kingdom, it always carries weight:

CHAPTER THREE - THE CREATOR'S MENU

* Eden's Test: The first sin entered through eating (Genesis 3).

* Israel's Consecration: Food laws shaped holiness (Leviticus).

* Daniel's Clarity: His diet sharpened his discernment (Daniel 1:8-17).

* The New Covenant: We remember Messiah through bread and wine (Luke 22:19-20).

This means what you consume is covenantal. Babylon says food is indulgence; Heaven says food is stewardship. Every meal is either obedience or compromise.

When you eat from the Creator's Menu, food becomes fuel for prophecy, prayer, and purpose. When you eat from Babylon's table, you dull your discernment, weaken your sensitivity, and shorten your stamina in consecration.

So ask yourself:

* Does what I put in my body create space for His presence?

* Does this meal align me with clarity, or clutter my spirit?

* Am I feeding my cravings, or am I feeding His calling?

Eating and drinking are worship, because worship is alignment. And when your appetite aligns with YAH's design, your body becomes more than a temple—it becomes an altar where His glory rests.)

Let's be clear—eating and drinking are never "just" physical. In the Kingdom, these are deeply spiritual acts:

They are acts of stewardship: When we eat, we are choosing how to care for the temple YAH (The LORD) has entrusted to us (1 Corinthians 6:19-20).

They affect spiritual clarity: What we consume impacts our energy, emotions, and ability to hear from The Ruach (The Spirit of God). Daniel's clarity increased when he ate according to conviction (Daniel 1:8-17).

They are tied to covenant: The first sin in Eden came through eating. The new covenant is remembered through eating (Luke 22:19-20). What we eat, and how we eat, matters to YAH (The LORD).

So when we say eating and drinking are spiritual—we mean they are part of how we honor, obey, and walk in intimacy with the Most High. Babylon calls it indulgence. Heaven calls it worship. Our choices are Kingdom declarations "Whether therefore ye eat or drink..." Paul names the most basic acts: eating and drinking. Why? Because how we treat the little things reveals what we truly value. Every bite we take is either obedience or indulgence, honor or habit. In the Reset, we learn: it's not just about what we consume—it's about why. Ask yourself, "Does what I put in my body make space for His presence?" Worship is a lifestyle, not a location "...or whatsoever ye do..." The glory of YAH (The LORD) isn't confined to church walls.

It shows up in how we speak, how we steward, how we move, how we eat. We must begin to see our entire lives—including our meals—as altars. Heaven doesn't separate sacred from physical—it sees alignment.

What you do in private (your plate, your pantry, your prayer life) prepares you for public power. The Goal is Glory "...do all to the glory of God." Everything we do should reflect back to the Father. Our reset is not about image—it's about imaging Him. The body is a temple. When we cleanse it, we invite greater glory. Eating to the glory of God means we choose what strengthens, not what weakens—what brings light, not what brings bondage. Ask yourself, "Is my lifestyle glorifying the One who made this temple?"

Closing Declaration:

"Father, reset my appetite. Not just for food, but for You. Let every bite, every drink, every act—bring You glory."

- *"I beseech you therefore, brethren, by the mercies of God, that ye present your bodies a living sacrifice, holy, acceptable unto God, which is your reasonable service."*—Romans 12:1

- *"And the very God of peace sanctify you wholly; and I pray God your whole spirit and soul and body be preserved blameless unto the coming of our Lord Yahusha HaMASHIACH (Jesus Christ)."*—1 Thessalonians 5:23

- *"Beloved, I wish above all things that thou mayest prosper and be in health, even as thy soul prospereth."*—3 John 1:2

A Prophetic Charge to the Remnant

If Babylon has fed you lies, then it's time to spit

them out of your mouth. If your temple has been desecrated, then it's time to consecrate. This isn't about food alone—it's about faith. This isn't about nutrition—it's about obedience.

The Garden was never closed. It was guarded. Through Yahusha HaMASHIACH (Jesus Christ), the sword has been lifted.

You now have access.

- Every fruit, eat with reverence
- Every herb, blend in wisdom
- Every seed, consume with thanks

It is a prophetic act. You're not just nourishing the body. You're rebuilding an altar. Let this not be a temporary fast—but a permanent shift. The reset isn't what you do. It's who you become.

CHAPTER THREE - THE CREATOR'S MENU

> Then Daniel said… "Test your servants for ten days; give us vegetables to eat and water to drink."
> – DANIEL 1:12

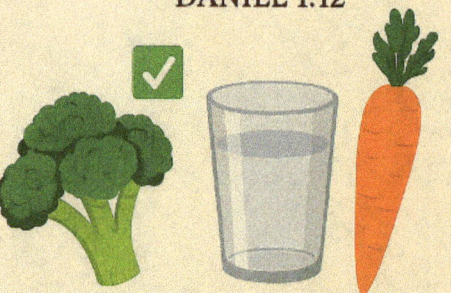

- Cleanse the body
- Clear the mind
- Consecrate the spirit

Chapter Four

The 7-Day Detox Blueprint
Resetting the Temple with intentionality

APPOINTED FOR THE RESET: A PROPHETIC INTRODUCTION

"Before I formed you in the womb I knew you, before you were born I set you apart; I appointed you as a prophet to the nations."

— *Jeremiah 1:5 (NIV)*

"Before I shaped you in the womb, I knew all about you. Before you saw the light of day, I had holy plans for you: A prophet to the nations."

— *Jeremiah 1:5 (The Message)*

The *Temple Reset* is a combination of personal experience shared through testimony, research-based evidence, scripture from wherever The Ruach Ha'Qodesh (Holy Spirit) has led me, and most importantly—obedience. This book was not born out of convenience. It was born out of divine commission.

In the process of walking out this Reset, I went to YAH (The LORD) for clarity—and He brought to light something He had already planted: I'm a trained Master Social Worker. Through that formal training, I learned about human development and the life cycle model. Through deliverance, spiritual maturity, and Kingdom calling, I learned how His eternal plan weaves through every stage of our journey. He led me to Jeremiah to understand how what was written then applies to us now.

Appointed by Yahuah (God, LORD, or Jehovah)

The word for YAH's (The LORD) people in this hour is clear: **Live a life of purpose on purpose.** We must be intentional. To reap the benefits of this Temple Reset—Detoxing our bodies, Renewing the Mind, Reclaiming the Spirit—we must understand that we were created with divine intent. You are who and what you are by purpose. Not in spite of yourself, but because of *whose* you are.

Yahuah (God, LORD, or Jehovah) is omniscient. He knew Jeremiah's strengths and weaknesses—and He knows ours. He knew we would possess exactly what He wants to use in these trying times. Some of us, like Jeremiah, have been set aside for special assignments revealed later in life. That's not just a coincidence. That's an *appointment*.

Though we may not all be prophets, we are all made in His image. The Word confirms it:

"Then God said, 'Let Us make man in Our image, in Our likeness, and let them rule over the fish of the sea and the birds of the air...'"

— Genesis 1:26

"For those God foreknew, He also predestined to become conformed to

the image of His Son... And those He predestined, He also called; those He called, He also justified; and those He justified, He also glorified." —*Romans 8:29–30*

There was an appointed time for your deliverance, also an appointed time for your works. The Ruach Ha'Qodesh (Holy Spirit) is a Gentleman. It is up to *you* whether or not you accept your divine assignment, just as it was for Jeremiah.

The 7-Day Detox Blueprint: Resetting the Temple with Intentionality

- *"Then Daniel said... 'Test your servants for ten days; give us vegetables to eat and water to drink.'"*

    —*Daniel 1:12*

This is not a diet. This is dominion. This is not about losing weight. It's about regaining alignment. The 7-Day Detox Blueprint is a spiritual act of obedience—a divine strategy to purify the temple and restore the rhythm of Heaven within us.

Each day is rooted in Kingdom principle and scriptural foundation. Each day offers an opportunity to:

1. Cleanse the body
2. Clear the mind
3. Consecrate the spirit

THE TEMPLE RESET

Day 1: Repentance & Reset

"Create in me a clean heart, O God, and renew a right spirit within me."—Psalm 51:10

* Morning: Lemon + ginger water for internal cleansing
* Journaling prompt: "What am I releasing today?"
* Prayer of repentance for neglecting the temple
* Food focus: Raw fruits + spring water. Today, your temple begins. Again—not in shame, but in surrender.

Testimony of Transformation: When I was hospitalized, I weighed 312 lbs. I didn't start this journey for weight loss, but three weeks after being released, I was 304. I began following the Temple Detox while increasing prayer, meditation, consecration, and fasting. Even though the weight loss was unintentional—it was welcomed. I noticed I could walk up the stairs without holding the banister or grunting. One day I put on a shirt that used to fit tight—I'd leave the bottom buttons undone. This time, it buttoned easily and looked marvelous. I stood sideways in the mirror and thought my eyes were playing tricks on me. No—it was evidence. For the first time in twenty years, I am under 300 lbs. YAH (The LORD) is healing temples; mine is one of them.

Day 2: The Mind Cleanse

"Be transformed by the renewing of your mind"

— Romans 12:2

* Morning: Detox Tea + Sea Moss Smoothie

CHAPTER FOUR - APPOINTED FOR THE RESET

* Reflection Prompt: "What thoughts need to be taken captive today?"
* Scripture Meditation: Read Romans 12:1-2 aloud
* Food focus: Steamed vegetables, avocado, seeds, and herbal tea
* Digital Detox: Limit media intake, increase worship and silence As your body detoxes, so must your thoughts. Let the Word rewire your perspective. The temple is not just physical—it's also mental.

Day 3: The Gut Reset

"Out of your belly shall flow rivers of living water."

— *John 7:38*

* Morning: Apple cider vinegar + warm water
* Food Focus: Fermented foods, high-fiber greens, flaxseed
* Reflection: What have I been spiritually and physically digesting?
* Prayer Focus: Healing for past trauma stored in the gut. The gut is not just the body's center—it's the seat of spiritual flow. Cleanse the river so it can flow freely.

Day 4: The Emotional Flush

"Cast your cares upon Him, for He cares for you."

— *1 Peter 5:7*

* Morning: Holy Basil or Ashwagandha Tea

- * Food Focus: Light broth, berries, greens
- * Journaling: What emotions am I holding that need releasing?
- * Practice: Take a walk and pray aloud. The body keeps score; so does the Spirit. Flush the pain. Make room for peace.

Day 5: Restoration & Strength

"They that wait upon the Lord shall renew their strength…"

— Isaiah 40:31

- * Morning: Protein smoothie (plant-based)
- * Food Focus: Chickpeas, lentils, quinoa, nuts
- * Movement: Gentle stretching or walking
- * Reflection: Where is YAH (The LORD) calling me to be stronger? You are not just being cleansed. You are being rebuilt.

Day 6: Spiritual Fire

"Is not My word like fire?" says the Lord

— Jeremiah 23:29

- * Morning: Ginger + cayenne detox shot
- * Food Focus: Anti-inflammatory foods (pineapple, turmeric, greens)
- * Worship: Extended time in praise
- * Prayer for Rekindling the Fire: Father YAH, I come before You as Your temple—open, willing, and ready. I ask

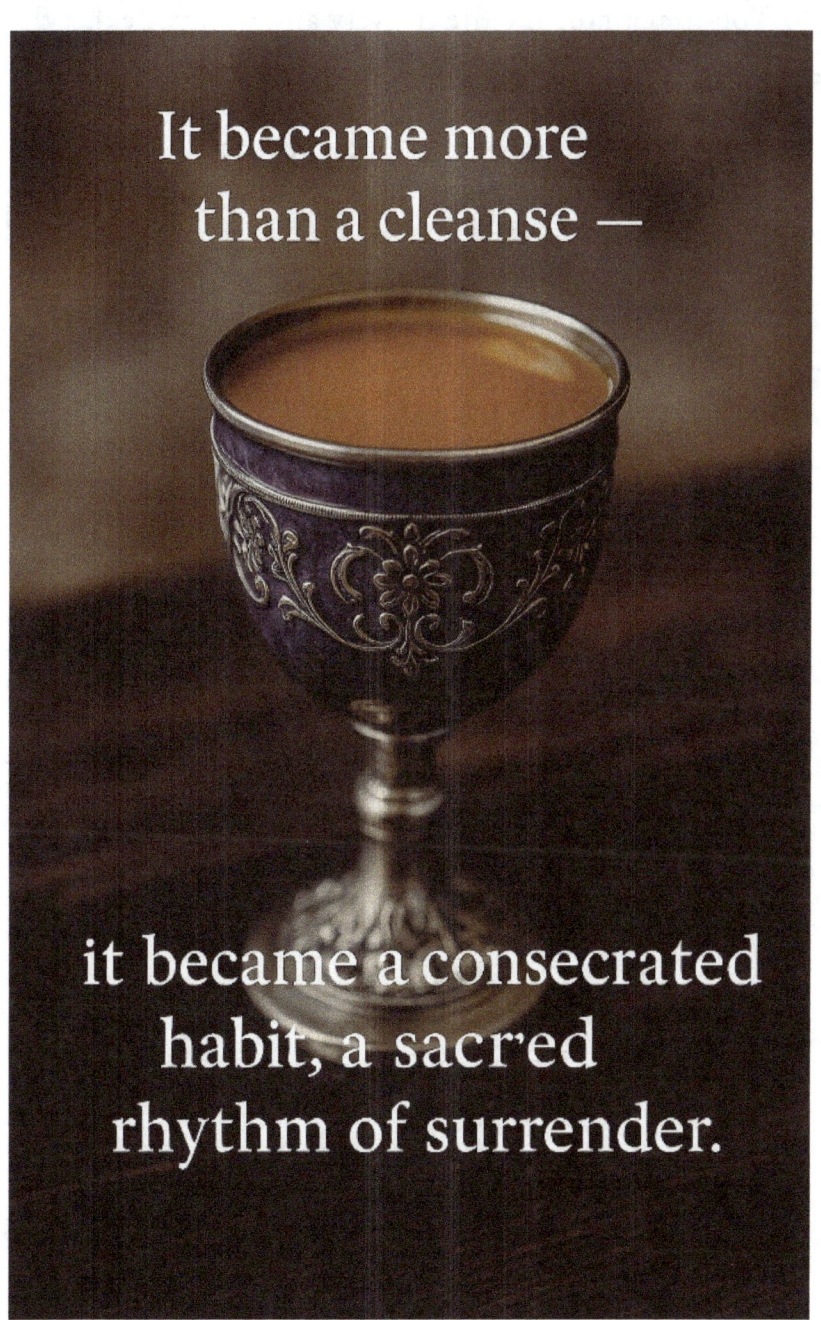

It became more than a cleanse — it became a consecrated habit, a sacred rhythm of surrender.

You to rekindle the fire in every area of my life. Let the embers that have grown cold be stirred again by Your Ruach. Detox my mind from confusion. Detox my heart from compromise. Detox my body from every unclean agreement I have made with Babylon. But don't let this detox stop at removal, Abba. Let it be renewal. Fill the empty spaces with Your presence. Replace weakness with strength, fear with faith, and dullness with fresh discernment. Let the fire fall! Let it consume what is not of You, and ignite everything that is. Set my altar ablaze with holiness, my voice ablaze with truth, my walk ablaze with obedience. Today I declare: I will not live lukewarm. I will burn bright for Your glory. I will walk renewed, refined, and revived.

In the name of Yahusha Ha'Mashiach (Jesus Christ)—Amein (Amen) and Amein (Amen).

Day 7: Consecration & Communion

"Present your bodies a living sacrifice..."

— Romans 12:1

* Morning: Coconut water or chlorophyll water
* Food Focus: Light, plant-based foods
* Activity: Rest and reflect
* Communion: End your fast with gratitude and sacred communion. You made it. You surrendered. You reset. Now go forth—restored, reconnected, and realigned.

CHAPTER FOUR - APPOINTED FOR THE RESET

The Elixir of Alignment: A Sacred Reset Drink

This isn't just a recipe—it's a ritual of obedience, a whispered warning against the war on our wellness, and a sacred strategy against generational dis-ease."

Temple Reset Recipes

"Taste and see that YAH (The LORD) is good."

— Psalm 34:8

These recipes are designed to support your 7-Day Detox journey and beyond, offering healing, cleansing, and nourishment—all rooted in the Creator's original design.

1. Morning Detox Drink (Shared Testimony Recipe)
2. The Elixir of Alignment: A Sacred Reset Drink
3. 1 fresh lemon (or lime, alkalizing alternative)
4. 1-inch piece fresh ginger, peeled and sliced
5. 12-16 oz warm spring water

Optional: pinch of cayenne pepper or raw honey

Instructions

1. Squeeze lemon or lime into warm water.
2. Add ginger and cayenne or honey if desired.
3. Stir, sip slowly in the morning before food. This drink I've laid out is like a backwoods apothecary revival—simple, natural, and potent. Let's break down how this elixir might help lower A1C, based on its ingredients

and what science has whispered over the years (since shouted truth often gets silenced):

1. Bragg's Apple Cider Vinegar (2 Tbsp)

The main player here. Multiple studies have shown apple cider vinegar (ACV) can improve insulin sensitivity and lower blood sugar spikes after meals. It may slow down carbohydrate digestion, which keeps glucose from spiking and helps the body process it more gradually. Regular intake (especially before meals) has been linked to lowering fasting blood glucose, which directly affects A1C levels.

2. Lemon Juice (1 Tbsp)

Rich in vitamin C and antioxidants, lemon may improve cellular response to insulin and reduce oxidative stress, both of which help control blood sugar. The acidity can also slow digestion, blunting blood sugar spikes.

3. Raw Honey (1 Tbsp)

Here's the odd duck. Raw honey is still sugar, but—unlike processed white sugar—it contains antioxidants, enzymes, and minerals. When used in moderation, it may cause less of a spike and can even have anti-inflammatory properties that benefit insulin sensitivity. That said, if A1C is already high, you might want to reduce to 1 tsp or eliminate altogether until levels stabilize.

4. Rosemary (1/16 tsp, boiled)

This herb has anti-diabetic properties, possibly enhancing insulin sensitivity and reducing blood glucose. Boiling it releases its essential oils and phenolic compounds, which are the good stuff. Also helps with inflammation and oxidative stress, which play a role in diabetes complications.

5. Turmeric (1/16 tsp)

Contains curcumin, which has powerful anti-inflammatory and blood-sugar-lowering properties. Can improve pancreatic function and increase glucose uptake in cells.

6. Cayenne Pepper (1/16 tsp)

Stimulates circulation and may help in reducing blood sugar levels by activating metabolism. Contains capsaicin, which may help regulate blood sugar in part by increasing insulin sensitivity.

The Method Matters

Boiling the rosemary activates its compounds. Letting it cool before adding ACV, lemon, and honey ensures you don't kill off the live enzymes and probiotics in the raw honey and ACV. Drinking it cold? That's just good sense—it likely tastes like righteous fire and lemony lightning.

So, how does it lower A1C? By:

1. Improving insulin sensitivity (ACV, turmeric, rosemary)

2. Reducing blood sugar spikes after meals (ACV, lemon, turmeric)

3. Combating inflammation (turmeric, rosemary, lemon)

4. Possibly improving digestion and metabolism (cayenne,

lemon, ACV)

Caution and Wisdom:

This isn't a magic potion, but more like a helpful foot soldier in the war against high A1C.

*Always check with your doc if you're on diabetes meds—ACV and turmeric can interact or intensify their effects.

Best consumed 15-30 minutes before a meal, especially a carb-heavy one. If used wisely, consistently, and as a part of a bigger lifestyle change, this drink might just nudge that A1C number down—like a gentle shepherd guiding wayward sheep back into the fold. *"This drink is how I started every morning during my detox. It became more than a cleanse—it became a consecrated habit, a sacred rhythm of surrender."*

Temple Smoothie: Green Fire

- 1 cup spring water or coconut water
- 1 tbsp sea moss gel
- 1/2 frozen banana
- 1/2 avocado
- 1/2 cup spinach
- 1/4 tsp spirulina powder
- 1/2 cup frozen pineapple

Instructions: Blend until smooth. Drink as a morning meal or energy reset.

Fire-Broth for Renewal

- 2 cups water
- 1/2 onion (sliced)
- 2 cloves garlic
- 1-inch ginger
- 1 tsp turmeric powder
- Dash of sea salt

Optional: cayenne for heat

Instructions:

1. Simmer for 15-20 minutes.
2. Strain and drink warm.

This broth supports digestion, detox, and clarity during fasting.

Stir-Fry Temple Bowl

- 1 tbsp avocado oil or coconut oil
- 1/2 cup broccoli florets
- 1/2 cup sliced bell peppers (any color)
- 1/4 cup red onion, sliced
- 1/2 cup zucchini or squash, sliced
- 1/2 cup cooked quinoa or brown rice
- 1 tbsp coconut aminos (soy-free alternative)
- 1/4 tsp turmeric

- 1/4 tsp ground ginger
- Pinch of sea salt
- Fresh cilantro or parsley for garnish

Instructions:

1. Heat oil in a skillet over medium heat.
2. Add onion and sauté for 2–3 minutes until soft.
3. Add remaining vegetables and stir-fry until tender but still vibrant.
4. Stir in turmeric, ginger, sea salt, and coconut aminos.
5. Serve over quinoa or brown rice and garnish with fresh herbs.

This dish is rich in fiber, antioxidants, and color—aligning your temple with vibrant life.

Chickpea Glory Bowl (Garbanzo Bean Stir Fry)

- 1 tbsp olive oil or avocado oil
- 1 cup cooked garbanzo beans (chickpeas)
- 1/2 cup cherry tomatoes, halved
- 1/2 cup chopped spinach or kale
- 1/4 red onion, thinly sliced
- 1 clove garlic, minced
- 1 tbsp coconut aminos or low-sodium tamari
- 1/2 tsp cumin

CHAPTER FOUR - APPOINTED FOR THE RESET

- 1/4 tsp paprika
- Pinch of sea salt and black pepper
- Squeeze of lemon or lime

Instructions:
1. Heat oil in a skillet over medium heat.
2. Add onion and garlic, sauté for 2-3 minutes.
3. Add chickpeas and seasonings. Stir well and cook for 5-7 minutes.
4. Toss in tomatoes and greens. Stir until wilted and heated through.
5. Finish with lemon or lime juice.

A perfect protein-packed, anti-inflammatory meal that satisfies without slowing the temple.

You might find the following resources helpful:

"Cleansing Therapy - Cure Yourself": This guide offers insights into detoxification and cleansing therapies.

thetempleofhealing.org

"Detoxification to Promote Health: A 7-Day Program": A comprehensive program focusing on detoxification to enhance health.

fammed.wisc.edu

Temple Ingredient Insights: Nutritional & Spiritual Value

- Spinach

Nutritional Value: High in iron, magnesium, vitamins A, C, and K

Spiritual Value: Symbolizes strength, clarity, and humility—leafy greens represent renewal

- Garlic

Nutritional Value: Natural antibiotic, anti-inflammatory, supports immune system

Spiritual Value: Drives out impurities—both in body and spirit. Often seen as a symbol of spiritual cleansing

- Sea Moss

Nutritional Value: Contains 92 of the 102 minerals the body needs; supports thyroid, digestion, and energy

Spiritual Value: Represents the abundance of Yah's (The LORD) oceanic provision and restoration

- Lemon & Lime

Nutritional Value: Detoxifying, alkalizing, high in vitamin C

Spiritual Value: Symbol of purification and divine clarity

- Olive Oil

Nutritional Value: Heart-healthy fat, anti-inflammatory, supports brain and joint health

Spiritual Value: Biblically symbolic of anointing and consecration

CHAPTER FOUR - APPOINTED FOR THE RESET

- Garbanzo Beans (Chickpeas)

Nutritional Value: High in protein, fiber, and essential vitamins

Spiritual Value: A symbol of provision, strength, and sustaining grace

- Quinoa

Nutritional Value: Complete protein, high in fiber, magnesium, and antioxidants

Spiritual Value: A "grain of promise"—sustaining for long journeys of faith

- Berries (Blueberries, Strawberries, etc.)

Nutritional Value: Rich in antioxidants, vitamins, and fiber

Spiritual Value: Represent sweetness in discipline—a reminder that obedience yields reward

- Ginger

Nutritional Value: Anti-inflammatory, aids digestion, boosts immunity

Spiritual Value: A root of fire and healing—ignites spiritual sharpness

- Turmeric

Nutritional Value: Contains curcumin, a powerful anti-inflammatory and antioxidant

Spiritual Value: Signifies healing and wholeness; a golden reminder of sanctification

These ingredients are not only tools of nourishment—they are testimonies. What you put into your body is also a way of declaring what you believe about who made it.

Healing Brown Rice Bowl

- 1 cup cooked brown rice
- 1/2 cup roasted sweet potatoes (cubed)
- 1/2 cup sautéed kale or collard greens
- 1/4 cup shredded carrots
- 2 tbsp pumpkin seeds
- 1 tbsp tahini or almond butter drizzle
- 1 tbsp fresh lemon juice
- Pinch of sea salt, black pepper, and smoked paprika

Instructions:

- Start with a warm bed of brown rice in a bowl.
- Layer sweet potatoes, greens, and carrots over rice.
- Sprinkle with pumpkin seeds.
- Drizzle with tahini or almond butter and lemon juice.
- Season lightly and serve warm.

This bowl brings grounding, fiber-rich nourishment—steadying both body and spirit.

CHAPTER FOUR - APPOINTED FOR THE RESET

THE TEMPLE RESET

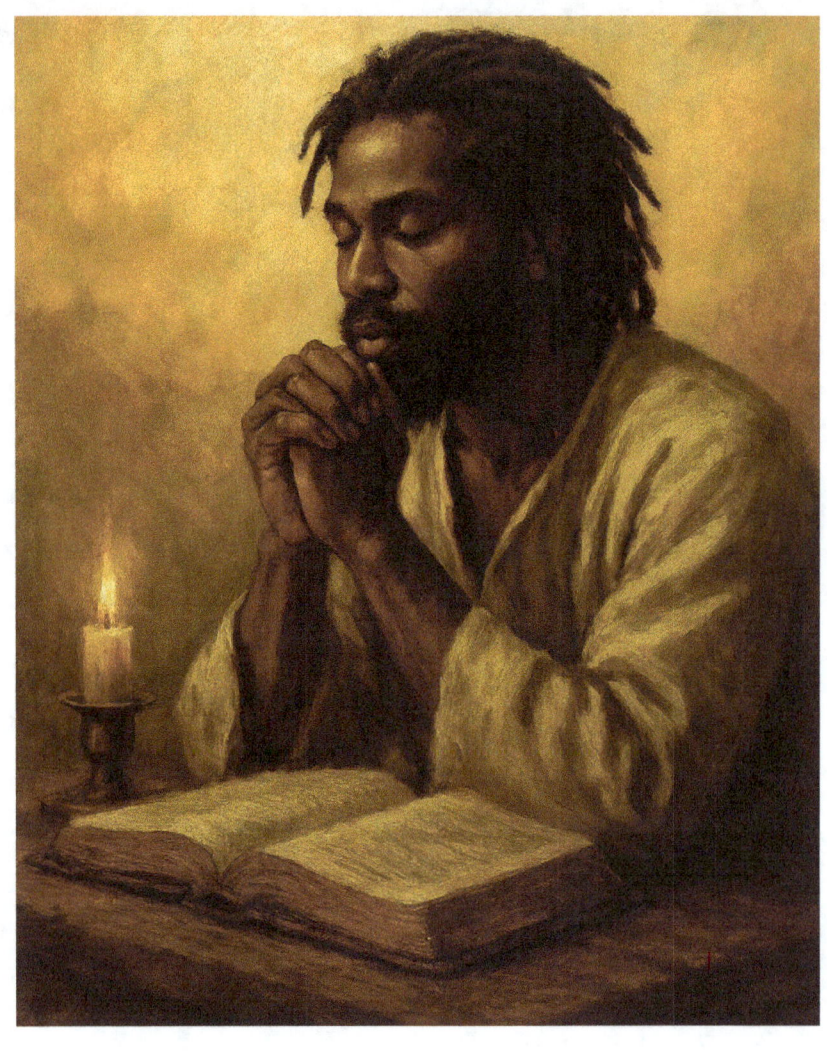

Chapter Five

DAILY DEVOTIONALS: MORNING & EVENING PRAYERS

"Let my prayer be counted as incense before you, and the lifting up of my hands as the evening sacrifice."

— Psalm 141:2

Consecration: Definition, Purpose & Benefits

Definition: Consecration is the act of setting oneself apart for sacred use. It means dedicating or devoting something exclusively to the Most High. In the Hebrew Bible, the word for consecrate is *qadash*, meaning "to sanctify," "to prepare," "to dedicate," or "to be holy."

"The Lord said to Moses, 'Say to the Israelites… Consecrate yourselves and be holy, because I am the Lord your God. Keep my decrees and follow them. I am the Lord who makes you holy.'"

—Leviticus 20:1, 7–8

Purpose: The purpose of consecration is alignment. It is a response to the call of YAH (The LORD) to live a life that reflects His holiness. It is about preparing ourselves to be vessels of honor, fit for the Master's use. Through consecration, we separate from the profane and draw nearer to the sacred. It is not just an act of ritual—it is a heart posture.

> *"Consecrate yourselves, for tomorrow the Lord will do amazing things among you."* —Joshua 3:5

Benefits of Consecration:

- Clarity of mind and spirit
- Increased sensitivity to The Ruach Ha'Qodesh (Holy Spirit)
- Strengthened spiritual authority
- Deliverance from strongholds
- Renewal of the mind
- Activation of gifts and callings

Greater intimacy with YAH (The LORD)

Consecration isn't something we do once. It's a rhythm—a lifestyle. Morning and evening devotions are the sacred rhythm of the Temple Reset. They remind us who we are, whose we are, and how we are to live.

For those walking deeper into maturity, this is not just about cleansing your outer life. It's about reaffirming the covenant that you shall have no other Elohim before Him. That nothing—not food, not fear, not ambition, not comfort—will be enthroned above YAH (The LORD). He alone is your Source, your Deliverer, your Life. This is for those who understand that the posture of your temple determines the presence you carry.

What True Devotion Looks Like in Action

True devotion is not simply what we say in prayer—it's how we posture our hearts and live our daily lives. It's seen in:

- The early riser who opens the day not with scrolling, but with scripture.
- The one who turns down a meal to feed the spirit in fasting.
- The person who guards their words, because their mouth is an altar.
- The one who walks away from a tempting conversation or habit, not in weakness but in worship.
- The believer who forgives again, prays again, surrenders again—because love is stronger than offense.

Devotion is discipline married to desire—it's loving YAH (The LORD) enough to make Him the center of your schedule, your habits, your body, and your choices. It is the fragrance of faith in motion.

"The Call to Consecration"

"Consecrate yourselves and be holy, because I am the Lord your God... I am the Lord who makes you holy."—Leviticus 20:1, 7-8

1. The Call is Personal—"Consecrate yourselves"

YAH (The LORD) doesn't consecrate us without

our consent. He initiates, but we must respond. Consecration begins with *intentional obedience*. This isn't about religious performance; it's about willingly surrendering what is common so YAH (The LORD) can make it holy.

Reflection: What am I holding onto that YAH (The LORD) is calling me to lay down?

2. The Standard is Holiness—"Be holy, because I am the Lord your God."

This is not a suggestion—it's a divine expectation. Holiness isn't about perfection. It's about proximity. The closer you walk with YAH (The LORD), the more like Him you become. Holiness is the fragrance of intimacy.

Reflection: Am I reflecting the holiness of the One I claim to walk with?

3. The Power is His—"I am the Lord who makes you holy."

You are not expected to consecrate yourself in your own strength. YAH (The LORD) is the one who does the sanctifying. Our job is to yield. His Spirit does the refining, the cleansing, and the renewing. We present the vessel—He purifies the temple.

Reflection: Am I relying on His power or my performance?

Morning Prayer Template

Heavenly Father, I rise to meet You with praise on my lips

CHAPTER FIVE - DAILY DEVOTIONALS

and gratitude in my heart. Thank You for breath in my lungs and strength in my body. Consecrate this day. Make my thoughts pure, my motives holy, and my actions aligned with Your will. Lead me by Your Spirit and help me honor You in all that I do. I yield my body, mind, and soul to You. Fill me with Your presence. Use me for Your glory. In the name of Yahusha HaMASHIACH (Jesus Christ), Amein (Amen).

Scripture of the Day: Ask YAH (The LORD) to lead you to a verse each morning and journal how it speaks to you.

Journaling Prompt: "What am I inviting into my temple today—and what must I cast out?"

Evening Prayer Template

Abba Father (Our Heavenly Father), Thank You for carrying me through this day. Forgive me for anything that grieved Your Spirit. Cleanse me from hidden faults and renew my strength. I lay down my worries, my weariness, and my thoughts. I receive Your peace. Speak to me in dreams and awaken me with purpose. Consecrate my rest. Let this night be holy unto You. In Yahusha's (Jesus) name, Amein (Amen).

Evening Reflection: "Where did I see the hand of YAH (The LORD) today?"

Journaling Prompt: "What did I learn today about YAH (The LORD), myself, or others?"

Let every prayer become incense. Let every breath be worship. Let every moment in His presence stir reflection, realignment, and responsibility. If you've read this far, then

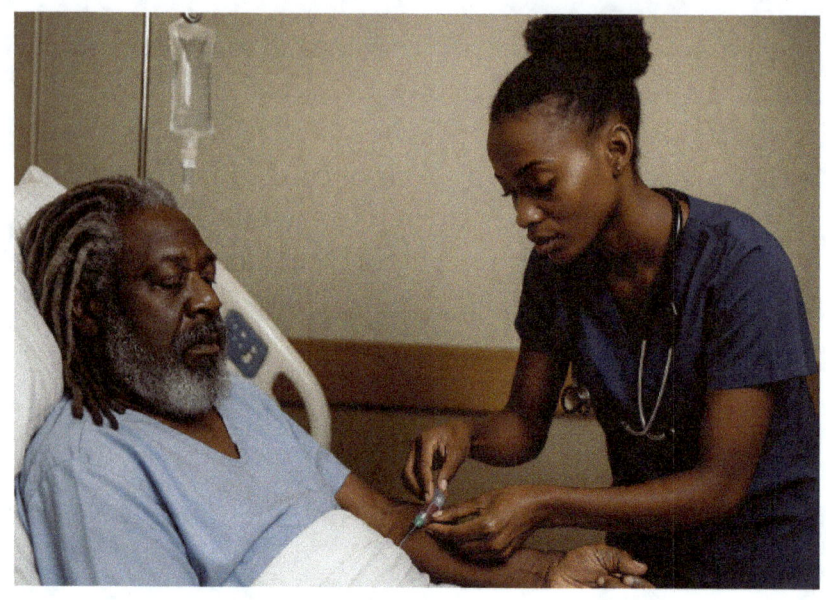

you know—this isn't just about devotion; it's about decision. Ask yourself: What is one thing I can surrender right now to draw nearer to YAH (The LORD)? Then do it today. Consecration isn't just a concept—it's a call. Now that you've heard it, what will you do with it? Let your devotion reshape your days—morning by morning, evening by evening—until your entire life becomes a sanctuary.

Personal testimony: when consecration reconnected me to the Most High.

Yah (The LORD) wants you to be yourself, not someone else. He wants your uniqueness to reflect His character. Look like you. Act like Him. Yah (The LORD) is love. He is: patient, kind, not envious, not boastful, not proud, not rude, not self-seeking, not easily angered, not a keeper of records of wrongdoing. He does not rejoice in evil, but He rejoices in the truth. Yah (The LORD) always

CHAPTER FIVE - DAILY DEVOTIONALS

protects, trusts, preserves. Yah (The LORD) never fails.

Yah (The LORD) wants us to express His nature: He wants us to "Be" versus "Look." Yah (The LORD) wants us to enjoy fellowship with Him. We can accomplish this through intentional daily devotion, worship, prayer, praise, and fasting. As I practiced the 7-day detox for two weeks, incorporating daily consecration, prayer, meditation, praise, worship, and fasting, I noticed that I even lost weight without trying. I was amazed to discover I weighed 297 lbs—under 300 for the first time in 20 years.

This transformation began with a divine disruption. I had fallen out of rhythm in January. The weight of grief from my son Maurice's birthday on January 4 led me to consume over ten pounds of sugar. My devotional life had fallen off. My blood glucose spiked to 767, and I was hospitalized. I had lost fellowship through disobedience, and the consequences were severe. Yah (The LORD), in His mercy, restored me.

The Ruach (The Spirit of God) stirred remembrance. My reconnection was a return to purpose. Until there is a reconnection between Yah's (The LORD) Ruach (Spirit of God) and man's spirit, we remain disconnected from our calling. Yah (The LORD) designed us for dominion over the earth—not for the earth to have dominion over us. Alcohol, drugs, and even sugar are signs of misplaced dominion.

The world around us is full of confusion, chaos, and lawlessness. Yah (The LORD) has appointed us—like Jeremiah—to uproot and tear down, to build and to plant. Our mission isn't just to deconstruct; it's to reconstruct in righteousness. It's time to live a life of purpose on purpose.

    I close with this: Yahusha (Jesus) is the Word manifested in the flesh. We are the flesh that is to be manifested in the Word. Let your temple tell the truth of who He is—not just by what you say, but by how you live.

CHAPTER FIVE - DAILY DEVOTIONALS

THE TEMPLE RESET

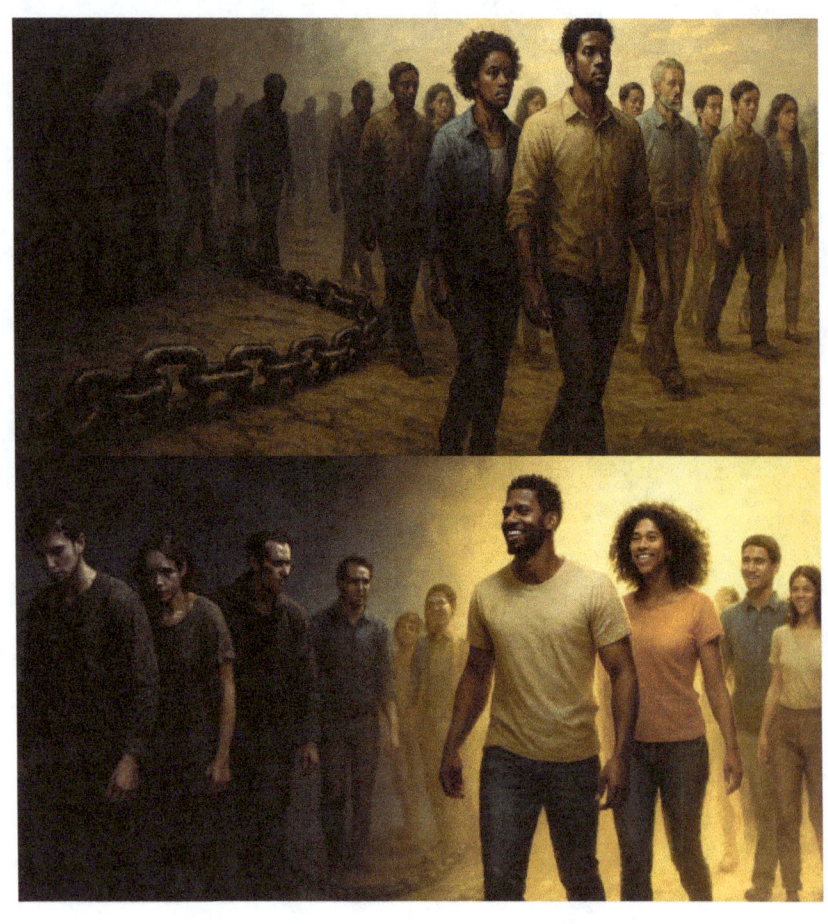

Chapter Six

BREAKING THE CHAINS OF BABYLON

---

1. Introduction: The Babylonian Blueprint

Babylon isn't just a city—it's a system. A masterclass in confusion, substitution, and seduction. It teaches us to trade the sacred for the synthetic and the eternal for the expedient. From the foods we eat to the days we worship to the hierarchies we unconsciously uphold, Babylon has infiltrated every corner of our consciousness. It's time to expose the blueprint, tear down the scaffolding, and return to the foundation.

The Most High is calling His remnant to shake off the spiritual amnesia and remember who we are and whose we are. Revelation 18:4 echoes like a trumpet: *"Come out of her, My people, lest you share in her sins, and lest you receive of her plagues."* This chapter is a reckoning. Not with the world alone, but with the systems we've accepted as normal.

2. Food as a Form of Control: Additives, Cravings & Chemical Chains

You are what you eat, they say. What if what we eat has been weaponized? From high-fructose corn syrup to artificial dyes, from GMOs (Genetically Modified Organisms) to chemical preservatives, the modern food system has done more than nourish—it's numbed. Spiritual clarity is dulled when the temple is defiled. Babylon's kitchen serves confusion, cravings, and compromise.

Scripture told us plainly: *"And God said, Behold, I have given you every herb bearing seed... to you it shall be for meat."* (Genesis 1:29). Instead of the Creator's menu, we've adopted a diet of addiction. Artificial additives alter our hormones, compromise our focus, and tether us to cravings that are spiritual as much as physical.

Returning to a Genesis-based lifestyle isn't just about diet—it's about dominion. Fasting, detoxing, and eating whole foods are forms of spiritual warfare. Babylon doesn't just feed the body; it manipulates the soul. We must reclaim what nourishes not just our flesh, but our faith.

3. The Sabbath Swap & Sacred Name Substitution

The seventh day Sabbath was never man's idea. It was YAH's (The LORD) sign of covenant, a day sanctified, set apart, and blessed. Somewhere between Constantine and convenience, man decided to edit God's calendar. The result? A Sunday swap cloaked in tradition, not truth.

CHAPTER SIX - BREAKING THE CHAINS OF BABYLON

Daniel 7:25 warned us: *"He shall intend to change times and law."* Babylon's fingerprints are all over this substitution. The Roman emperor Constantine legalized Christianity and outlawed Sabbath observance in favor of Sun-day worship—a nod to pagan sun-gods, not the Son of God.

This doctrinal overhaul was codified in events like the **Council of Nicaea (325 AD)**, which not only reshaped the calendar but also defined orthodoxy according to imperial agenda. The **Council of Trent (1545–1563)** later doubled down, affirming Sunday worship as a mark of the Church's authority and declaring tradition equal to Scripture.

It didn't stop there. The names of the Father and the Son were also swapped, filtered through Greek and Latin tongues, stripped of their Hebrew identity. *YHWH* became "the LORD." *Yahusha* or *Yeshua* became "Jesus." What was holy was renamed to fit the narrative of the empire. Names carry identity, authority, and covenant. To reclaim the name is to reclaim the nature.

Honoring the Sabbath is not legalism; it's loyalty. It's not a ritual; it's relationship. When we restore the rhythm of reverence and call upon the true Name, we align with divine order. Coming back to Sabbath—and to sacred names—is a prophetic protest against Babylon's calendar and counterfeit language.

4. Social Stratification: The Babylonian Ladder

Babylon loves to divide. Race, class, gender, status—its strength lies in separation. Social stratification is not just a cultural issue; it's a spiritual strategy. The Tower of

THE TEMPLE RESET

Babel was man's monument to himself, a vertical hierarchy that reached to the heavens but ignored heaven's heart.

In this present day, that tower still stands—in corporations, churches, governments, and gated communities. The illusion of superiority is Babylon's most successful export. YAH (The LORD) is no respecter of persons. The Kingdom does not function on ladders but on love. The remnant must reject the hierarchy and embrace the humility of Messiah, who washed feet instead of climbing ranks.

5. Institutionalized Inequality: Religion, Education, and Economic Manipulation

Babylon doesn't just create systems; it creates cages. Religion without revelation. Education without elevation. Economics without equity. The beast system has embedded injustice into the very institutions we're told to trust.

Pulpits have become platforms for popularity, not prophecy. Schools teach us how to pass tests but not how to test spirits. Financial systems reward exploitation over stewardship. It's all rigged to keep the masses malnourished—physically, mentally, and spiritually.

The Kingdom is rising. A people who will no longer be spoon-fed deception. A people who will read, research, and return to the truth.

6. Reclaiming the Truth: A Remnant Rises

The remnant is awakening. No longer content with religion draped in Roman robes or food baptized in chemicals. This is the season of discernment. We must test every teaching, trace every tradition, and challenge every chain.

CHAPTER SIX - BREAKING THE CHAINS OF BABYLON

The road back to Eden is narrow, but it is marked by truth. Repentance, re-education, and reformation are the tools of this remnant. The call is not to reform Babylon but to exit it. In our exodus, we find Eden.

7. Prayers of Repentance & Reconciliation

Father, forgive us for trading Your truth for tradition. For calling what is holy common, and what is common holy. We repent for eating what defiles, for worshiping on days You did not sanctify, and for submitting to systems that oppress Your image in us. We repent also for forsaking Your sacred Name and replacing it with the titles and inventions of man.

Restore our hunger for righteousness. Teach us to detox not just our bodies, but our beliefs. Lead us back to Your order, Your timing, and Your truth. Let us call upon Your Name in spirit and in truth.

We renounce the chains of Babylon and embrace the liberty of Your Kingdom.

8. Evidence-Based Research & Resources

(see the Resources)

9. Final Charge & Reflection Questions

Final Charge: Babylon's spell is subtle but strong. It lulls us into comfort, conformity, and compromise. You were not made for its chains. You were born to be a temple of Yahuah (God), set apart, awakened, and walking in truth. Break free. Burn the lies. Bless the Name. Then, walk in the authority of the Kingdom. You are not just escaping Babylon—you're helping others find their exodus too.

Reflection Questions:

1. What areas of your life still operate under Babylon's influence?

2. Have you adopted traditions that conflict with scriptural truth? What are they?

3. In what ways has your diet affected your spiritual clarity?

4. What steps can you take this week to begin detoxing your body, mind, and spirit?

5. How can you help others awaken to these truths without condemning them?

6. What name do you call upon—and does it reflect the truth of your covenant with the Most High?

7. How do church councils like Nicaea and Trent influence your current understanding of doctrine?

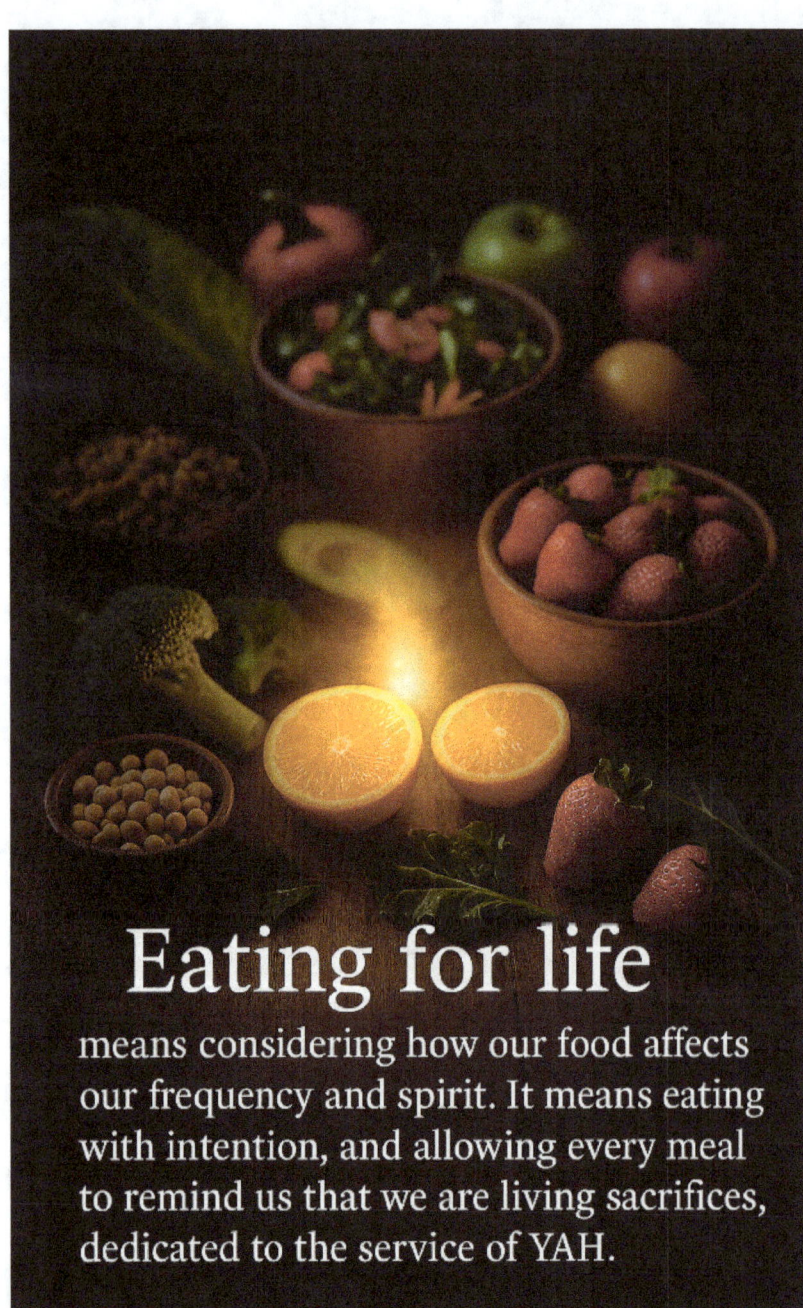

Eating for life

means considering how our food affects our frequency and spirit. It means eating with intention, and allowing every meal to remind us that we are living sacrifices, dedicated to the service of YAH.

Chapter Seven

AFTER THE RESET—HOW TO EAT FOR LIFE

1. Introduction: From Deliverance to Discipline

The detox is done. The fast has broken the grip. The temple has been reset. Now what? The wilderness always follows deliverance. After Egypt, there was the desert. After detox, there is discipline. The same grace that brought you out must now guide you in.

This chapter isn't just about what to stop eating—it's about how to start living. We move from what to remove to what to restore. From cleansing to covenant. From restriction to rhythm. Eating according to the Creator's design isn't a temporary fix—it's a lifestyle rooted in reverence, stewardship, and sanctification.

THE TEMPLE RESET

2. Returning to the Creator's Menu

Genesis 1:29 was not a suggestion; it was a blueprint. *"Behold, I have given you every herb bearing seed... to you it shall be for meat."* This original instruction wasn't lost—it was left. Buried under centuries of tradition, empire cuisine, and religious compromise.

Now we dig it back up. Fruits, vegetables, grains, nuts, seeds—living food for a living temple. This isn't just about going plant-based; it's about going purpose-based. Understanding the function of food: to heal, to energize, to build—not to pacify or destroy.

3. The Spiritual Frequency of Food

Everything in creation emits a frequency—every plant, every body, every breath. The Creator spoke the world into existence with sound, and sound is vibration. Frequency is the language of the spirit realm. When we eat foods that are alive, we tune our bodies to the rhythm of life, to the resonance of heaven.

Raw fruits, fresh vegetables, seeds, and herbs vibrate at high frequencies because they come straight from the source—untouched, unprocessed, unpolluted. In contrast, highly processed, microwaved, chemical-laden foods vibrate at low or even zero frequency, robbing the body of vitality and disrupting the spirit's sensitivity.

The human body, when healthy, vibrates around 62-72 MHz. Disease starts when the body drops below 58 MHz. Fear, bitterness, and junk food lower frequency. Worship, prayer, laughter—and yes, whole living foods—lift it.

CHAPTER SEVEN - AFTER THE RESET - HOW TO EAT FOR LIFE

Eating becomes an act of spiritual alignment. When we eat foods the Most High created in the form He intended, our temple resonates with His design. Our prayers gain clarity. Our dreams return. Our discernment sharpens. Spiritual fog begins to lift.

This isn't new-age nonsense—it's ancient wisdom. Daniel's choice to refuse Babylon's food was a frequency decision. He chose what would amplify his connection with YAH (The LORD), and the result was revelation, strength, and supernatural insight. When you eat light, you walk in light. The food you choose can either raise your discernment or bury your destiny.

4. Rebuilding the Altar: Eating as Worship

Every meal is a moment to honor the Most High. To pause. To pray. To thank Him for what was grown, not manufactured. This is more than nutrition; it's communion.

Blessing your food is not superstition—it's sanctification. The altar has shifted from stone to stomach. We are the priests now. What we place on the plate is our offering.

5. Practical Patterns for Lifelong Eating

Seasonal Eating: Align with the Creator's natural rhythm.

Intentional Fasting: Build fasting into your weekly or monthly routine for spiritual clarity and physical reset.

Meal Prep with Purpose: Plan with reverence, not convenience.

Label Discernment: Read every label like a Berean reads

Scripture—test every ingredient.

Hydration as Holy Habit: Water is living. Drink it like you believe it.

6. Freedom, Not Legalism

This is not about bondage to rules—it's about walking in wisdom. You are not under law but under love. Love disciplines. Love chooses what's best, not just what's easy.

Let no one judge you for where you start. Don't settle either. Keep moving toward holiness in every habit—including how you eat.

7. The Ministry of the Table

The table is a place of fellowship, healing, and remembrance. It's where Yahusha (Jesus) broke bread, taught truth, and shared presence. It is also where He revealed that betrayal was close—*"The one who dips his hand with Me in the bowl will betray Me."* (Matthew 26:23)

This wasn't just a place of peace; it was a place of prophetic revelation. What happens around the table has the power to expose, to restore, and to prepare. When we eat with purpose, we honor that legacy.

We must restore the sacredness of the table. Too often, meals have become isolated events—plates taken to bedrooms, heads bowed, not in prayer, but over screens. Attention given to devices rather than to one another. This is Babylon's blueprint: distraction, division, and disconnection.

Reclaim your table. Eat together. Share stories. Pray

CHAPTER SEVEN - AFTER THE RESET - HOW TO EAT FOR LIFE

aloud. Laugh. Cry. Talk about the Most High. Teach your children while they chew. Let your home echo the rhythm of righteous fellowship. The family that eats together doesn't just stay together—they grow together.

Open your table to others. Share what you've learned. Teach through your lifestyle. Because the reset isn't just for you—it's for your house, your circle, your community.

8. Closing Reflection & Charge

Your temple has been reset. Your appetite has been reclaimed. Now eat like someone who knows who they are. Don't go back to Egypt. Don't return to Babylon's buffet. Let your food be your faith in action. Let your plate preach. Let every bite be a testimony. You've been delivered. Now live delivered.

9. Prayer of Dedication

Father YAH (The LORD), Creator of all living things, Thank You for opening our eyes to what defiles and what sanctifies. Thank You for calling us back to Your table, to Your Word, to Your way. We dedicate our appetites to You. We surrender our cravings and our culture-conditioned habits. Cleanse our palates and our spirits.

Teach us to eat with honor, to prepare with prayer, and to serve with joy. Let our homes become sanctuaries of health, love, and truth. Let the table be where heaven meets earth, where unity is restored, and where You are glorified.

We declare: We will eat for life. We will live what we believe. We will not be slaves to Babylon's buffet. We are Your people, and this temple is Yours.

In the name of Yahusha (Jesus), the Bread of Life—Amein (Amen).

10. Reflection Questions

- What habits have you formed around food that may reflect Babylon's influence more than YAH's (The LORD) design?
- How can you begin to reintroduce the sacredness of the table in your daily life?
- Are you consuming food that lifts your frequency or lowers it? What needs to change?
- How does your eating reflect your spiritual walk? What does your plate say about your priorities?
- In what ways can you invite your family and community to journey with you into eating for life?
- Have you asked the Father to sanctify your appetite? If not, what's stopping you?

CHAPTER SEVEN - AFTER THE RESET - HOW TO EAT FOR LIFE

THE TEMPLE RESET

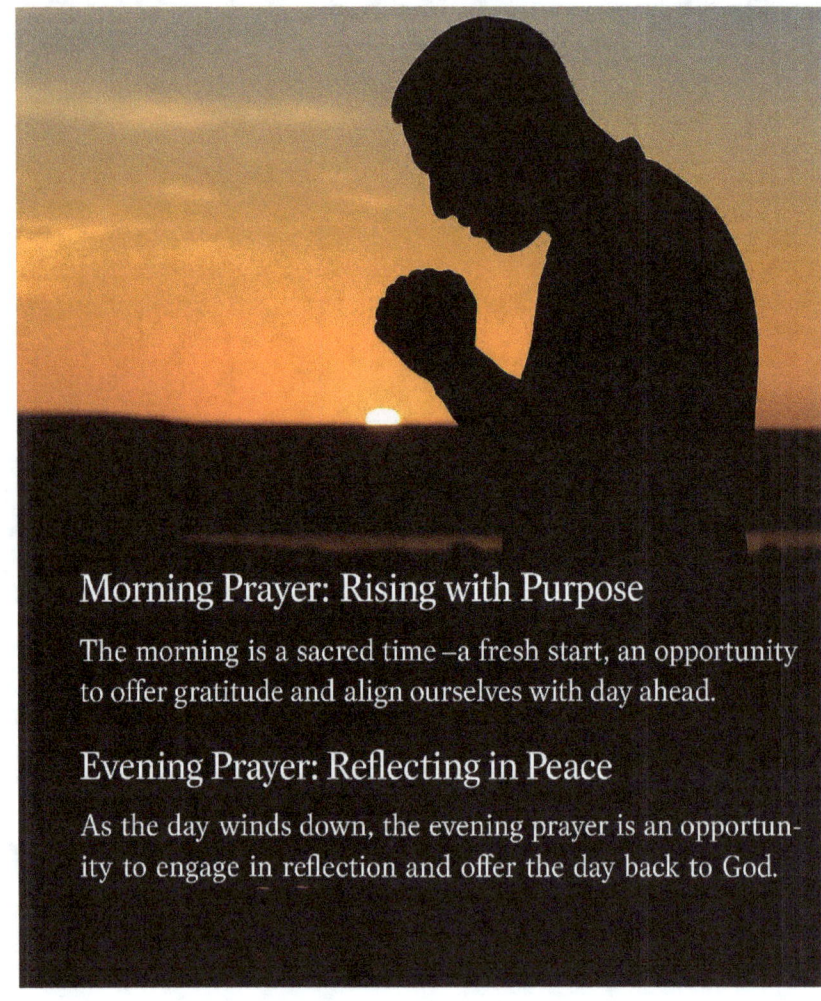

Morning Prayer: Rising with Purpose

The morning is a sacred time –a fresh start, an opportunity to offer gratitude and align ourselves with day ahead.

Evening Prayer: Reflecting in Peace

As the day winds down, the evening prayer is an opportunity to engage in reflection and offer the day back to God.

Chapter Eight

DAILY DEVOTIONALS:
MORNING & EVENING PRAYERS (PT. 2)

---

1. Introduction: Bookends of the Day

Just as the sun rises and sets by divine appointment, so too should our days begin and end in fellowship with the Most High. Morning and evening prayers aren't just religious routines, they are sacred rhythms. They center us. They reset us. They frame our daily battles in eternal truth.

The world trains us to reach for our phones first and collapse into bed last. The Kingdom teaches us to rise with purpose and rest with peace. These prayers are not filler—they're fire. Morning ignites your mission; evening seals your soul in Shalom (Peace).

2. Morning Devotional: Aligning with the Assignment

Scripture Meditation: *"This is the day which YAH (The LORD) has made; we will rejoice and be glad in it."* – Psalm 118:24

Prayer: ABBA YAH (God the Father), As I offer myself to You, do with me as You will. Provide relief from the flaws of me that I may do good work by which others see and glorify You. Thank You for awakening me to another day of purpose. I surrender this day to You—my thoughts, my actions, my interactions. Let Your Word be the lamp to my feet and the light to my path.

Sanctify this temple afresh. Cleanse my motives. Guide my conversations. Let me walk in humility and boldness, clothed in righteousness and truth. Let me see interruptions as divine appointments, and challenges as opportunities to glorify You.

I put on the full armor of YAH (The LORD). Let no weapon formed against me prosper. Let my words be seasoned with grace and my heart anchored in Your promises. Lead me beside still waters, and restore my soul throughout this day.

This is Your day. Use me for Your glory. Amein (Amen).

3. Midday Devotional: Reset and Refocus

Scripture Meditation: *"He restores my soul: He leads me in the paths of righteousness for His name's sake."* – Psalm 23:3

Prayer: Father YAH (The LORD), At the midpoint of this day, I pause to realign with You. Quiet the noise around me and within me. Let Your Spirit steady my focus and recharge my purpose.

Where I've drifted, redirect me. Where I've fallen, forgive me. Where I've succeeded, keep me humble. Let me finish strong—anchored in truth, led by Your Ruach (Spirit of God).

Reignite my energy, renew my joy, and remind me why I began today with You. Let the second half of this day bring You even more glory than the first. Use me for Your glory.

In Yahusha's (Jesus) name—Amein (Amen).

4. Evening Devotional: Returning to Rest

Scripture Meditation: *"I will both lay me down in peace, and sleep: for You, YAH (The LORD), only make me dwell in safety."* – Psalm 4:8

Prayer: Father YAH (The LORD), Thank You for sustaining me through this day. I return to You tonight with a heart of gratitude. Thank You for protection, provision, and correction. Even in the things I didn't understand, You were present.

I lay down every worry, every failure, every unfinished task. I release offense. I forgive and ask to be forgiven. Search me, O YAH (The LORD), and know my heart. Purge anything unclean. Wrap me in Your Shalom (Peace) as I sleep.

Renew my spirit. Restore my joy. Recalibrate my purpose. Let my dreams be visions from You, and my rest be holy.

I trust You with my breath, my body, and my tomorrow. In

Yahusha's (Jesus) name—Amein (Amen).

5. Weekly Sabbath Devotional: Entering His Rest

Scripture Meditation: *"Remember the Sabbath day, to keep it holy."* - Exodus 20:8

Prayer: ABBA YAH (God the Father), We enter this Sabbath with reverence and rest. Thank You for this set-apart time, a holy pause to remember who You are and who we are in You. Cleanse our hearts of busyness and burdens. Fill our homes with peace and praise.

Let this day be a sanctuary in time. Let our conversations be edifying. Let our meals be simple and sacred. Teach us to delight in this rest, not as obligation, but as invitation.

May the Sabbath restore what the week has drained. May Your presence dwell richly among us.

We honor You, YAH (The LORD), in our rest. We honor You in our rhythm. Amein (Amen).

6. Consecration Prayer: Fasting & Spiritual Warfare

Scripture Meditation: *"Is not this the fast that I have chosen? To loose the bands of wickedness, to undo the heavy burdens..."* — Isaiah 58:6

Prayer: YAH (The LORD) of Hosts, In this season of consecration, we set aside every earthly appetite for the pursuit of Your presence. We fast not for attention, but for alignment. We strip away distractions and silence the noise. Let Your voice be the only one we follow.

CHAPTER EIGHT - DAILY DEVOTIONALS (PT. 2)

Break every chain. Undo every lie. Uproot every idol. Let this fast be fire that purifies, not just abstinence, but transformation. Strengthen us where we are weak. Fill us with supernatural clarity and holy fire.

We reject the patterns of this world and embrace the power of Your Kingdom. Let angels be dispatched. Let strongholds be shattered. Let purpose be birthed. This fast is Yours. We are Yours. In Yahusha's (Jesus) name—Amein (Amen).

7. The Power of Rhythm

Morning and evening devotion anchor the believer. Just as the priests lit the lamps in the tabernacle day and night, so we kindle our flame through intentional prayer. This rhythm trains the spirit, disciplines the flesh, and welcomes The Ruach Ha'Qodesh (Holy Spirit) into the daily details. In Babylon, distraction is default. However, in the Kingdom, devotion is our weapon.

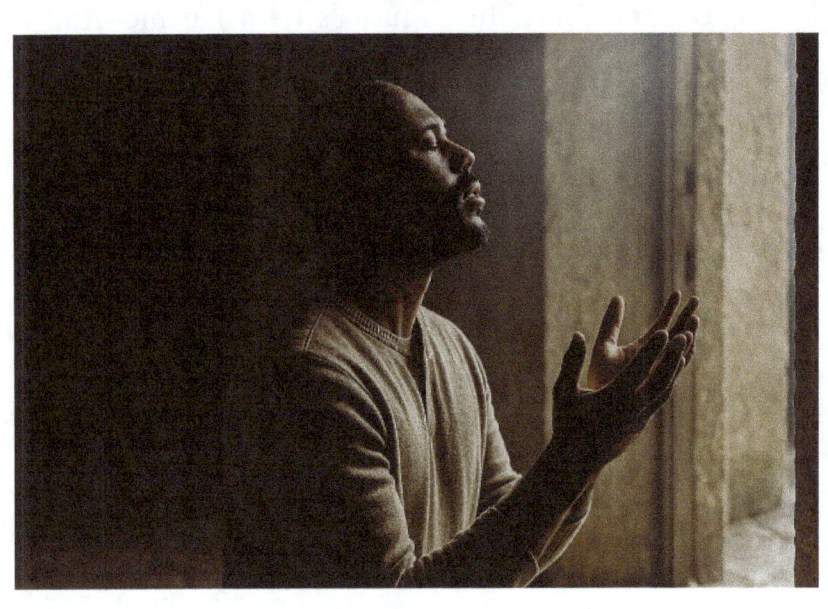

Chapter Nine

TEMPLE PRAYERS FOR PURIFICATION

---

1. Introduction: A Holy Cry from a Cleansed Temple

Prayer is not performance—it's purification. It's not recitation—it's relationship. When the temple is clean, the cry becomes clear. Our words carry weight not because of their length or eloquence, but because of the condition of the heart from which they rise.

This chapter gathers prayers for personal and collective purification—prayers that wash, consecrate, realign, and reawaken. These are not formulas but flames. They're meant to be prayed with fire, not only repeated with form. Pray them aloud. Write them in your journal. Cry them in your secret place. Let the altar of your heart burn again.

2. Prayer of Heart Purification:

YAH (The LORD), examine me and expose me. Search the corners of my heart and show me what I've justified but never repented of. Burn away what offends You. Purge every hidden idol. Dismantle every excuse.

Let my motives be sanctified. Let my thoughts be pure. Cleanse me from the inside out. Strip away the performance, the people-pleasing, the fear, and the pride.

Create in me a clean heart, O YAH (The LORD), and renew a right spirit within me. I want to walk in truth, live in light, and love without hypocrisy. In Yahusha's (Jesus) name—Amein (Amen).

Reflection:

- What has YAH (The LORD) revealed in your heart today?
- Are there excuses you've made that now require repentance?

3. Prayer of Tongue and Thought Purification

Abba (Father), I surrender my mouth and my mind. Forgive me for every idle word, every bitter complaint, every carnal thought. Cleanse my imagination. Sanctify my speech. Let my tongue become a tool of truth, not a weapon of destruction.

Let the meditations of my heart and the words of my mouth be acceptable in Your sight, O YAH (The LORD), my strength and my Redeemer.

CHAPTER NINE - TEMPLE PRAYERS FOR PURIFICATION

Guard my gate. Transform my thinking. Help me to be quick to listen, slow to speak, and slower still to wrath.

Let my mind be stayed on You. Amein (Amen).

Reflection:

- What recent words or thoughts do you need to bring under YAH's (The LORD) authority?
- How can you guard your speech and imagination today?

4. Prayer for the Purification of the Assembly

Most High, we come as a unified people, not only individualy. Cleanse Your Bride. Purify Your Body. Expose the mixture, the compromise, the entertainment, and the ego that have crept into Your house.

Restore reverence to Your sanctuary. Raise up leaders who fear You more than they fear crowds. Sweep through our pulpits, our pews, our programs.

Let repentance flood the altar. Let righteousness rise like incense. Purify us, that we may be holy as You are holy.

Let judgment begin at the house of YAH (The LORD)—and let mercy triumph over judgment. In the name of the Risen King Yahusha (Jesus)—Amein (Amen).

Reflection:

- How can you personally help restore reverence to the assembly?

- What compromises in the Body grieve your spirit?

5. Prayer of Daily Consecration

Abba Father (Our Heavenly Father), This day belongs to You. I set myself apart. Let my life be an offering. Let my habits be holy. Let my thoughts be disciplined and my time be guarded.

Keep me from distraction and deception. Let me not chase platforms but pursue Your presence. Let my private life reflect the purity I proclaim in public. I dedicate my hands, my feet, my voice, and my choices to You. Let me decrease, that You may increase. I am Yours—set apart, sealed, and sent,

In Yahusha's (Jesus) name Amein (Amen).

Reflection:

- What distractions do you need to surrender today?
- What area of your life needs deeper consecration?

6. Prayer of Repentance

YAH (The LORD) Elohim (God), I come not with excuses, but with honesty. I have sinned against You—in thought, word, and deed. I have turned from Your commands and followed my own counsel. Today, I return.

Forgive me for grieving Your Spirit. Wash me in the blood of the Lamb. Let the tears I cry extend beyond emotion. Let them be but transformational.

I renounce every agreement I made with darkness—know-

CHAPTER NINE - TEMPLE PRAYERS FOR PURIFICATION

ingly or unknowingly. Break the soul ties. Cancel the curses. Restore what rebellion cost me.

I fall into Your mercy. I rise in Your grace. In Yahusha's (Jesus) name—Amein (Amen).

"If my people, which are called by my name, shall humble themselves, and pray, and seek my face, and turn from their wicked ways; then will I hear from the heavens, and will forgive their sin, and will heal their land," says Yahuah Elohiym. II Divrei Hayamiym Sheniy (Deev-ray Ha-yah-meem Sheh-nee) Cepher."

If my people, which are called by my name, shall humble themselves, and pray, and seek my face, and turn from their wicked ways; then will I hear from heaven, and will forgive their sin, and will heal their land." 2 Chronicles 7:14 (KJV)

You are Yahuah (God, LORD, or Jehovah) who makes all things new.

Reflection:

- What sins do you need to specifically confess?
- What agreements with darkness must be broken today?

7. Prayer of Restoration

Restorer of the breach, Builder of ruins, Thank You for not leaving me in my brokenness. You are the God who makes all things new. Rebuild what was lost through disobedience. Reclaim what the locusts have eaten.

Restore my joy. Renew my strength. Reignite my purpose. Let me no longer be defined by what I did—but by who I'm becoming in You.

Make beauty from these ashes. Turn my mourning into dancing. Cover me with Your favor like a robe.

I receive full restoration by faith. Amein (Amen).

Reflection:

- What do you believe YAH (The LORD) wants to restore in your life?
- How will you walk in that restoration starting today?

8. Priestly Prayer of Intercession

Father of compassion, I stand in the gap for those who can't pray for themselves. For the weary, the wounded, the wandering, and the waiting: I plead the blood of Yahusha (Jesus) over every lost sheep, every backslider, and every prisoner of the lie.

Break chains today. Heal minds. Awaken spirits. Visit sons and daughters with dreams. Provoke fathers and mothers with repentance.

Let the prodigals return. Let the intercessors arise. Let revival begin in the hidden places. Use me as a vessel, to cry out and reach out. Not just to pray, but to love. In the name of the Great High Priest—Yahusha (Jesus) the Messiah—Amein (Amen).

CHAPTER NINE - TEMPLE PRAYERS FOR PURIFICATION

Reflection:

- Who has YAH (The LORD) placed on your heart to intercede for today?

- How can you be the vessel He uses in someone else's breakthrough?

THE TEMPLE RESET

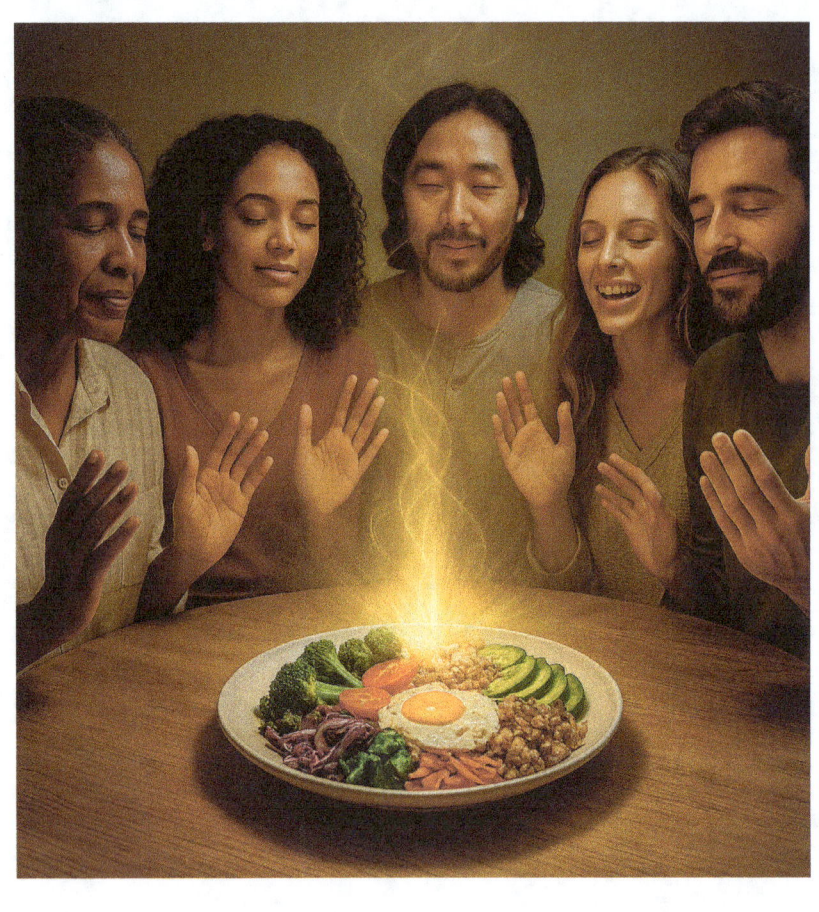

Chapter Ten

THE SPIRITUAL SCIENCE OF FOOD— HOW WHAT YOU EAT AFFECTS YOUR FREQUENCY

---

1. Introduction: Feeding the Flesh vs. Fueling the Spirit

Food has never been neutral. From the forbidden fruit in Eden to the King's meat in Babylon, what we consume has always carried spiritual consequences. We've been taught to count calories—but heaven counts the cost. Food doesn't just feed your body, it fuels or fogs your spirit.

YAH (The LORD) designed the human temple with divine intelligence. Every cell, every organ, every system is meant to work in harmony with His creation. Babylon's food system is filled with artificial additives, lab-grown confusion, and frequency-killing toxins.

This chapter reveals the science behind the scripture. How what you eat affects your body's electrical frequency—and how that frequency affects your discernment, clarity, and connection to the Spirit.

2. What Is Frequency, and Why Does It Matter?

Everything in creation vibrates. Everything. The universe, your body, your thoughts, even your food.

Frequency is the measurable rate of electrical vibration. Healthy humans typically vibrate at 62–72 MHz. But processed foods, artificial ingredients, and sugar-heavy diets lower that frequency fast—often into ranges that open the door for disease (and spiritual disconnection).

High-frequency foods (raw fruits, vegetables, herbs, seeds) vibrate with life. Low-frequency or "dead" foods (processed meats, fried items, microwave meals, artificial sweets) vibrate with decay.

The Kingdom operates on a higher frequency. The more you align with creation, the more you attune to the Creator.

3. Daniel's Diet: A Frequency Fast

Daniel 1:8–20 shows us what happens when someone refuses Babylon's buffet. Daniel and his companions abstained from the king's defiled food and drank only water, eating pulse (seeds, legumes, vegetables). The result?

CHAPTER TEN - THE SPIRITUAL SCIENCE OF FOOD

Greater wisdom, sharper appearance, and ten times the insight of all the magicians and astrologers.

Daniel wasn't only abstaining from food, he was fasting frequency interference. The clarity he received prepared him for prophecy, intercession, and elevation.

4. The Mind-Body-Spirit Connection

The temple is one unit. The mind, body, and spirit are not isolated. What affects one, influences the others. Brain fog, fatigue, depression, anxiety, and spiritual apathy are often connected to what we're putting into our mouths.

Spiritual apathy is a state of indifference, numbness, or lack of passion toward the things of Yahuah (God, LORD, or Jehovah). It's when a believer goes through the motions of faith—praying, attending service, reading Scripture—but without genuine fire, hunger, or devotion.

Scripture tells us to *"be transformed by the renewing of your mind."* That transformation doesn't stop with thoughts; it extends to biology. When your body is inflamed, your spirit is distracted. When your gut is toxic, your discernment dims.

When your temple is clean, the connection is clear. You hear YAH (The LORD) easier. You dream more vividly. You pray with authority. You walk lighter.

5. Foods That Heal, Foods That Hinder

High-Frequency, Healing Foods:

- Raw fruits and vegetables (especially leafy greens, berries, citrus)
- Sprouted grains and seeds
- Herbs (basil, oregano, cilantro, parsley)
- Cold-pressed oils (olive, flaxseed, hemp)
- Pure spring water

Low-Frequency, Harmful Foods:

- Refined sugars and high-fructose corn syrup
- Artificial colors, flavors, preservatives
- Processed meats and fast food
- Soda and sugary drinks
- GMO and pesticide-laden produce

6. **Detoxing Babylon's Buffet**

The reset requires release. You cannot walk in Kingdom power while feeding on Babylon's crumbs. Start with awareness—read your labels, ask questions, research ingredients. Then move to action—replace one dead food at a time with something that brings life.

Fasting is a frequency reset. A time to realign with YAH (The LORD), reset your physical cravings, and reawaken spiritual hunger.

7. Fasting Guide: Types and Purposes

Scriptural Fast Types:

- **Daniel Fast:** vegetables, water, and seed-based foods only (Daniel 1)
- **Complete Fast:** abstaining from all food for a time (Esther 4:16, Acts 9:9)
- **Sunrise to Sunset Fast:** no food during daylight (Judges 20:26)
- **Water-Only Fast:** deeply spiritual and physically demanding—seek Ruach's leading.

Fasting Purposes:

- To break yokes (Isaiah 58)
- To humble the soul (Psalm 35:13)
- To sharpen spiritual discernment (Acts 13:2-3)
- To detox and discipline the flesh (1 Corinthians 9:27)

Practical Tips:

- Fast with intention. Don't just stop eating—start seeking.
- Pair fasting with worship, journaling, and stillness.
- Break the fast gently with high-frequency foods.

8. Scripture Reflections: Frequency and Holiness

- **1 Corinthians 10:31** - "Whether therefore ye eat, or

drink, or whatsoever ye do, do all to the glory of God."

- **Isaiah 58:6** - "Is not this the fast that I have chosen..."
- **Psalm 104:14** - "He causeth the grass to grow for the cattle, and herbs for the service of man..."
- **Romans 12:1–2** - Present your bodies as a living sacrifice, transformed by the renewing of your mind.
- **3 John 1:2** - "Beloved, I wish above all things that thou mayest prosper and be in health, even as thy soul prospereth."

9. The Body as an Instrument of Worship

Romans 12:1 reminds us to *"present your bodies a living sacrifice, holy, acceptable unto God, which is your reasonable service."* That includes how you treat it, what you feed it, and how you keep it clean.

This body is not your own—it's His. So we don't eat for entertainment. We eat for energy, clarity, and covenant.

10. Final Thoughts: Eat with Eternity in Mind

This isn't about fear—it's about freedom. Babylon wants you addicted, sluggish, and spiritually dulled. YAH (The LORD) wants you alive, alert, and anointed. Let your food serve your faith. Let your plate preach. Let your appetite be ruled by the Spirit, not by the system.

When you eat light, you live light. When you eat life, you walk in Life. When you fuel your temple with

CHAPTER TEN - THE SPIRITUAL SCIENCE OF FOOD

what the Creator intended, you become a vessel that vibrates with truth, clarity, and Kingdom frequency.

Research Spotlight: Dietary Truths Confirmed

Many of the prophetic insights encountered earlier are supported by the following scientific studies. Here are key findings that affirm how diet impacts spiritual clarity, stamina, and mind renewal:Research Spotlight: Dietary Truths Confirmed

Many of the prophetic insights we encountered earlier are now supported by scientific studies. Here are key findings that affirm how diet impacts spiritual clarity, stamina, and mind renewal:

Research Finding Implication for Temple Reset

SMILES Trial (2017) - Dietary intervention with a whole-food, Mediterranean-style plan significantly reduced depressive symptoms compared to social support alone. Shows that changing food can change mood, clarity, and energy—essential for prayer stamina and spiritual sensitivity.

Ultra-Processed Foods & Depression (JAMA Network Open, 2023) High consumption of processed foods is strongly linked with higher risk of depression; these foods dull discernment and undermine spiritual fortitude.

Gut-Brain Axis Review (Cryan & Dinan, 2019) The gut microbiome sends signals to the brain — both for uplift and deterioration. What you eat shapes that line of spiritual communication.

MIND/Mediterranean Diets & Cognitive Health (2015) Diets rich in plants, whole grains, nuts, with low processed food intake are linked to slower cognitive decline and sharper thinking.

Inflammation & Ultra-Processed Foods (hs-CRP markers) Elevated inflammation is associated with poor diet; inflammation impairs cognition, energy, emotional stability — all required for sustained spiritual consecration.

Takeaway:

- These studies don't just support what the Spirit has already warned — they provide a roadmap.
- Let our eating become sober and intentional.
- Let our plates reflect our prayers.
- Let our diet not only sustain our bodies but sharpen our prayers, restore our clarity, and lengthen our consecration. Selah

CHAPTER TEN - THE SPIRITUAL SCIENCE OF FOOD

THE TEMPLE RESET

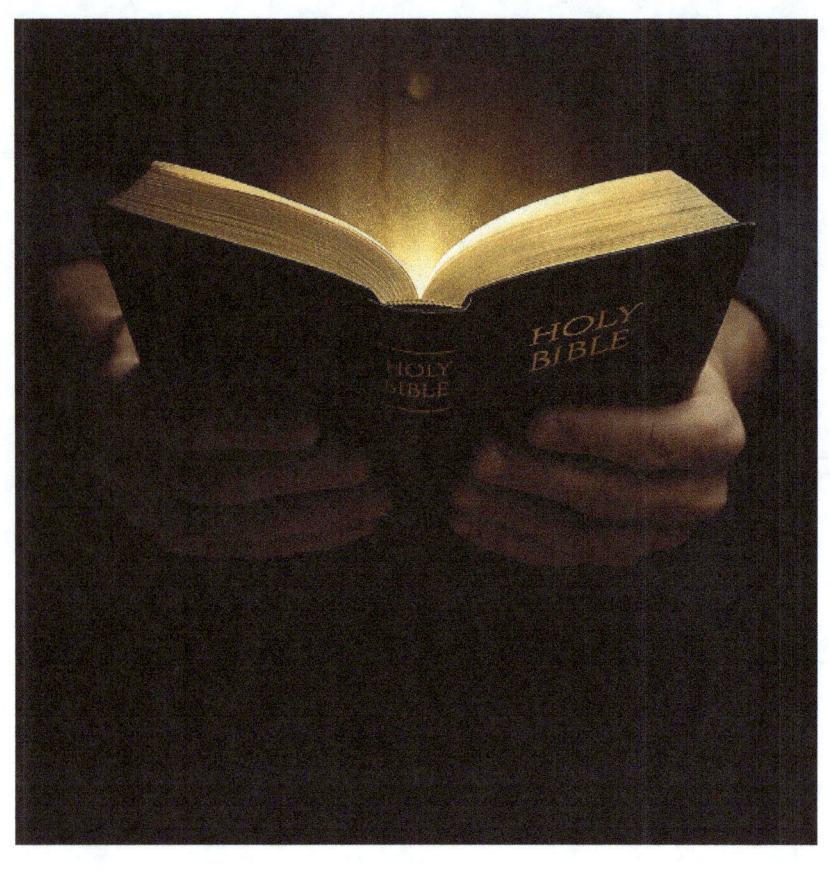

CHAPTER ELEVEN

SCRIPTURES FOR DELIVERANCE & HEALING

1. Introduction: His Word Is the Medicine

In a world of synthetic cures and temporary bandages, the Word of YAH (The LORD) remains the only medicine that heals at the root. Deliverance doesn't begin in a hospital—it begins in the heart. Healing doesn't start with pills—it starts with promises.

This chapter is not commentary. It's not a devotional. It is weaponry. *For the weapons of our warfare are not carnal, but mighty through God to the pulling down of strong holds.*—2 Corinthians 10:4

These scriptures are not to be passively read—they are to be declared, believed, and warred with. Speak them aloud. *So then faith comes by hearing, and hearing by the word of YAH.*—Romans 10:17

Meditate on them. Memorize them. Pray them over your body, your family, and your atmosphere.

The same Word that created your body is the Word that can restore it. *In the beginning was the Word, and the Word was with God, and the Word was God.*—John 1:1 *And the Word was made flesh, and dwelt among us... full of grace and truth.*—John 1:14

2. Scriptures for Physical Healing

- *Exodus 15:26*—"For I am YAH that healeth thee."
- *Isaiah 53:5*—"By His stripes we are healed."
- *Psalm 103:2–3*—"Who forgiveth all thine iniquities; who healeth all thy diseases."
- *Jeremiah 30:17*—"I will restore health unto thee, and I will heal thee of thy wounds."
- *James 5:14–15*—"And the prayer of faith shall save the sick, and YAH shall raise him up."

3. Scriptures for Deliverance from Bondage

- *John 8:36*—"Whom the Son sets free is free indeed."

- *Psalm 34:17*—"The righteous cry, and YAH (The LORD) heareth, and delivereth them out of all their troubles."

- *Colossians 1:13*—"Who hath delivered us from the power of darkness."

- *Luke 10:19*—"Behold, I give you power... over all the power of the enemy."

- *2 Corinthians 10:4*—"For the weapons of our warfare are not carnal, but mighty through God."

4. Scriptures for Emotional and Mental Healing

- *Isaiah 26:3*—"Thou wilt keep him in perfect peace, whose mind is stayed on thee."

- *Philippians 4:6–7*—"And the peace of God...shall keep your hearts and minds."

- *2 Timothy 1:7*—"For God hath not given us the spirit of fear."

- *Proverbs 17:22*—"A merry heart doeth good like a medicine."

- *Psalm 147:3*—"He healeth the broken in heart, and bindeth up their wounds."

5. How to Use These Scriptures in Your Walk

- **Pray them out loud daily**—activate the Word over your life.

- **Write them on sticky notes**—place them where your eyes go often.

- **Fast and meditate**—let the Word wash over weak or wounded areas.

- **Share with others**—healing flows through testimony and teaching.

6. Sample Healing Prayer

Father YAH (The LORD), I come to You as my Creator, Healer, and Redeemer. You formed me in the secret place, and You know every cell, every ache, every imbalance. I speak Your Word over this temple: By Your stripes, I am healed. I receive the healing purchased by Yahusha's (Jesus) sacrifice.

Let every system in my body align with Your design. Remove all disease, inflammation, and dysfunction. Let my mind be at peace, my emotions be stable, and my heart be whole. Touch me from the inside out and let healing manifest in Your perfect timing.

I trust You. I thank You. I glorify You. Amein (Amen).

7. Daily Deliverance Declaration

Today, I declare: I am not bound. I am free. I am not weak. I am filled with power. I am not a victim. I am more than a conqueror.

In Yahusha's (Jesus) name, I renounce every lie of the enemy, every generational curse, every soul tie, every spirit of fear, infirmity, or confusion.

I command my body, mind, and soul to come under the authority of the Most High. I plead the blood of Yahusha (Jesus) over every doorway of my life. This is my exodus. This is my restoration. This is my declaration. Amein (Amen).

8. Final Charge: Take the Prescription

Declare these scriptures not as hope—but as *truth*.

Speak them until your body obeys. Speak them until your soul aligns. Speak them until strongholds break. Because His Word never returns void.

9. Deliverance Self-Check Checklist

Use this checklist to prayerfully identify areas where deliverance may be needed. Mark the ones that apply and bring them before YAH (The LORD) in fasting and prayer:

- Repeated cycles of sin despite repentance
- Chronic fear, anxiety, or nightmares
- Unexplained sickness or heaviness
- Uncontrollable anger or emotional outbursts
- Addictions (food, sex, alcohol, media, etc.)
- Generational patterns of dysfunction or abuse
- Unforgiveness or bitterness that won't break
- Feelings of spiritual oppression or darkness
- Difficulty reading Scripture or staying in prayer
- Ongoing confusion or mental torment

If you've marked multiple areas, begin a season of intentional consecration, and ask for spiritual counsel and covering as needed.

10. Healing Testimony Page

Use this space to record what YAH (The LORD) has done

CHAPTER ELEVEN - SCRIPTURES FOR DELVERANCE & HEALING

for you. Your testimony will strengthen your faith and help set others free.

Date: _____

What did YAH (The LORD) heal or deliver you from?

What scriptures became real to you in this process?

How has your walk changed since the breakthrough?

Who have you shared your testimony with?

Final Praise: Write a prayer or declaration of thanksgiving to YAH (The LORD) below:

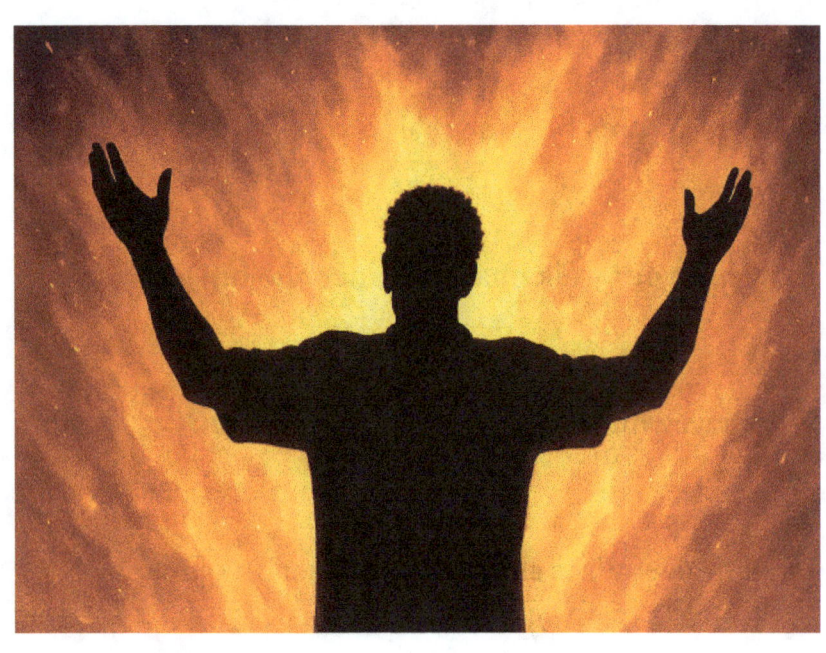

Chapter Twelve

THE GOVERNMENT OF HEALING — A CONSUMING FIRE FINALE

The Foundation of Governmental Order: Spiritual Gifts and the Way of Love

Before diving into the divine order of healing and holy government, we must anchor ourselves in how The Ruach Ha'Qodesh (Holy Spirit) distributes power and presence within the Body. Sha'ul's (Paul) words to the believers in Qorinth (Corinth)—preserved here from the Cepher—set the tone for the spiritual balance of power, purpose, and love:

QORINTIYM RI'SHON (1 CORINTHIANS) 12–13 (CEPHER)

Now concerning spiritual gifts, brethren, I would not have you ignorant. You know that ye were Gentiles, carried away unto these dumb idols, even as ye were led. Wherefore I give you to understand, that no man speaking by The Ruach Elohiym (Spirit of God) calls YAHUSHA (Jesus) accursed: and that no man can say that YAHUSHA (Jesus) is ADONAI (Lord), but by The Ruach Ha'Qodesh (Holy Spirit).

[Excerpt continues through 1 Corinthians 13]

"And now abides faith, hope, love, these three; but the greatest of these is love."

1. The Power of Twelve: Divine Government, Order, and Completion

In the language of the Spirit, numbers are never random. Twelve is the number of divine government, perfect order, and spiritual completeness. It's the structure that supports authority and releases alignment. From the twelve tribes of Israel to the twelve apostles of the Lamb, YAH (The LORD) has always moved through divine patterns.

QORINTIYM RI'SHON (1 CORINTHIANS) 14–15 (CEPHER)

Follow after love and desire spiritual gifts, but rather that ye may prophesy...

But now is MASHIACH (Messiah) risen from the dead and become

CHAPTER TWELVE - THE GOVERNMENT OF HEALING

the firstfruits of them that slept...

From Gifting to Governing: A Call to Maturity

We've read the fullness of Sha'ul's (Paul) revelation—not as theory, but as a charge. These chapters are a blueprint for a Body in transition: from scattered to synchronized, from gifted to governed, from fragmented to functioning in one Spirit.

The Ruach Ha'Qodesh (Holy Spirit) does not move randomly. He moves through assignment. Through structure. Through unity. Unity is not uniformity—it's harmony. Each gift, each role, each part of the Body must know its place, not for recognition, but for reconciliation. Heaven's government flows when earth's obedience responds.

This is the hour to stop competing and start completing. To stop flexing gifts and start building altars. We aren't just "vessels." We are extensions of His Kingdom. Apostles must honor prophets. Teachers must yield to truth. Healers must serve in humility. Every gift, every grace, must bow to the government of love. We were never meant to impress; we were meant to impart.

2. A Consuming Fire Finale: Refined by Love, Aligned by Spirit

This was never about gifts alone—it was about government. Government without love is tyranny. The Spirit's gifts were never meant to elevate men; they were meant to edify the Body. The Body cannot be edified where there is no order, no unity, and no love.

Sha'ul's (Paul) letters not only teach, they calibrate. They align our posture, our priorities, and our purpose. Every gift given by The Ruach Ha'Qodesh (Holy Spirit) is part of YAH's (The LORD) holy infrastructure, a spiritual system designed to heal individuals, and govern healing through love.

That's why this chapter closes with resurrection. Once the Body is aligned, once the temple is reset, once love becomes law, resurrection life flows.

This isn't just about healing the sick. It's about raising the dead things in our ministries, families, and personal walks. It's about watching what once laid dormant begin to breathe again.

It all points back to the Father. Every gift, every tongue, every prophecy, every miracle, every healed wound, every restored soul—points upward.

Let this chapter be your altar. Let the consuming fire of YAH (The LORD) burn up everything that's out of order and light up what was left in the dark. Because love never fails, and His government shall have no end. Amein (Amen).

Conclusion: The Reset Was the Beginning

The detox was never about diet alone. The frequency shift was never just about food. The purification was never just about your body. This entire journey—every chapter, every fast, every prayer, every revelation—was about bringing the temple back under divine government.

CHAPTER TWELVE - THE GOVERNMENT OF HEALING

You are not who you were. You have been called, cleansed, and commissioned. You've broken soul ties with Babylon. You've reclaimed the Creator's design. You've chosen purpose over pleasure, truth over tradition, and fire over familiarity. Nevertheless, this is not the end. This is the entrance. Now comes the stewardship. Now comes the lifestyle. Now comes the witness.

Walk in this reset—not as a trend, but as a testimony. Let your life prove that YAH (The LORD) still rebuilds ruins. Let your walk declare that holiness is still the standard. Let your temple be a sanctuary for His glory. **When the temple is clean, the fire will fall.** And the world will know it was Him all along.

Amein (Amen) and Amein (Amen).

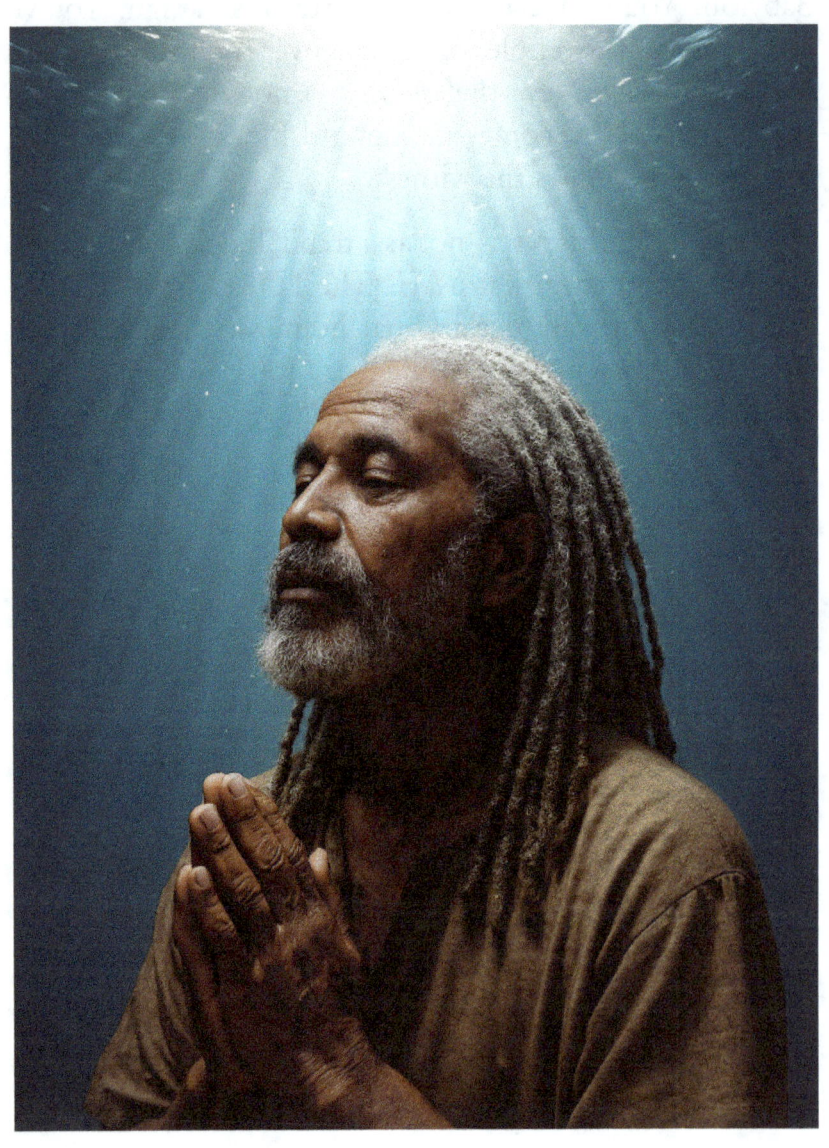

BONUS

The Temple Reset Workbook
(Condensed Companion Edition)

Introduction: More Than a Workbook—It's a Walk Back to the Father

This is not just a workbook. This is your altar. Your mirror. Your blueprint.

Each page has been crafted to take the teachings of *The Temple Reset* and turn them into transformation. Every reflection, every prayer, every prompt is designed to help you interact with YAH (The LORD), not just the words on the page. The goal is not perfection—it's *presence*.

THE TEMPLE RESET

Whether you're walking through this journey alone, with a small group, or leading a ministry, this workbook is here to help you:

- Anchor your identity in the Creator's original design

- Break agreements with systems that defile the temple

- Cultivate healing through discipline and devotion

- Step into Kingdom alignment and spiritual maturity

Each section is synced to the corresponding chapters in *The Temple Reset* and includes:

- **Key Scriptures**

- **Personal Reflection Prompts**

- **Group Discussion Questions**

- **Prayer Focuses**

- **Action Steps**

BONUS SECTION — COMPANION WORKBOOK

- **Testimony & Tracking Pages**

There's also space for fasting notes, frequency shifts, and daily realignment.

You don't need a degree to walk in holiness. You need obedience, humility, and Ruach-led rhythm. Use this workbook like a compass. May it point you back to the Father, again and again.

When the temple is clean, the fire will fall.

Let's walk it out.

Amein (Amen).

[Chapters 1-12 Companion Reflections Here - Condensed as per printed book formatting. Full edition available separately.]

Testimony Page

- Before this reset, I was...

- During the reset, I learned...

- After the reset, I am...

- I give YAH (The LORD) all the glory because...

Scripture Memorization Tracker Write and recite one scripture per week that strengthens your temple walk.

- Week 1: _____

- Week 2: _____

- Week 3: _____

- Week 4: _____

- Bonus Verses: _____

7-Day Fasting & Frequency Journal Record what you eat, how you feel, and what you hear in the Spirit.

- Day 1: _____

- Day 2: _____

- Day 3: _____

- Day 4: _____

- Day 5: _____

- Day 6: _____

- Day 7: _____

Morning Devotional Template

- Scripture of the Day: _____

- Prayer: _____

- What I'm Thankful For: _____

- Today I will honor the temple by: _____

Evening Devotional Template

- What YAH (The LORD) revealed today:

THE TEMPLE RESET

_____

- What I need to release: _____

- Prayer of Surrender: _____

Weekly Reset Reflection Page

- What victories did I walk in this week? _____

- What still needs resetting? _____

- What is The Ruach (The Spirit of God) saying for the week ahead? _____

- Where do I need to submit more deeply? _____

Group Leader's Guide: Leading a Temple Reset Study

Purpose: To guide a group of believers through *The Temple Reset* with clarity, conviction, and community.

Leader Tips:

BONUS SECTION — COMPANION WORKBOOK

- Open and close every session with prayer.

- Encourage vulnerability but protect confidentiality.

- Stay rooted in Scripture, not opinion.

- Be flexible—let Ruach lead, not the clock.

- Provide space for journaling and testimony.

Weekly Group Flow:

1. **Welcome + Prayer (5–10 min)**
2. **Reflection & Check-In (15–20 min)**
3. **Scripture & Workbook Discussion (30–40 min)**
4. **Action Step + Closing Prayer (10–15 min)**

Suggested Tools:

- Printed workbooks or notebooks

- Bibles with restored names (if available)

- A clean space for fellowship—no distractions

Closing Encouragement To the leaders, intercessors, and shepherds—thank you for saying yes. You're not just hosting a study. You're stewarding a movement. Every session is an altar. Every heart is sacred ground. Every breakthrough belongs to YAH (The LORD).

Keep pointing them to the Father. Keep modeling the message. Because when the fire falls, they'll remember the vessel who lit the match.

Amein (Amen) and Amein (Amen).

ABOUT THE AUTHOR

From an injured mess to a Messenger, Pastor Wright does not consider himself a "religious man." Rather, a man of covenant, by the power of the Ruach Ha'Qodesh (Holy Spirit), His life and work flow out of a personal relationship with Yahusha HaMashiach (Jesus Christ). To him, this is the same Redeemer many have encountered; Brian simply chooses to honor the Sacred Hebrew Name, the fruit of his journey to study and show himself approved.

This author's calling is to point others beyond tradition [ritual] and into truth, [relationship]. His writing, music, and ministry all carry one consistent thread: restoring the covenant path and lifting the Name above every name.

Through Anointed Recorded Ministers Industry (ARMI LLC) and Transformation Ministries Inc., Brian carries out this mission globally—publishing, teaching, and equipping the remnant of Yahuah's people to walk in truth, wholeness, and spiritual authority.

GLOSSARY

ABBA YAH (Ahb-bah Yah) (commonly known as God the Father)—Teaches intimacy and reverence for Yahuah as our covenant-keeping Father.

Abba Father (Ahb-bah Fah-ther) (commonly known as Our Heavenly Father)—Reveals the closeness of a child's cry—"Abba"—to the Creator of all.

Adonai — (Lord, Master)

Amein (Ah-main) (commonly known as Amen)—Affirms agreement with Yahuah's word, meaning "so be it" in truth.

Babylon (Bah-bah-lawn) (commonly known as The World/system opposed to God)—Represents rebellion, corruption, and the counterfeit systems of man.

Elohiym (El-oh-heem) (commonly known as God)—Highlights the Mighty One, Creator of heaven and earth.

Hamaschiach / HaMASHIACH (Ha-mah-shee-akh) (commonly known as The Anointed One, The Christ)—Points to the consecrated Savior, set apart to redeem mankind.

MASHIACH (Mah-shee-akh) (commonly known as Messiah, Christ)—Declares the promised Deliverer of Israel and the world.

Ruach Elohiym (Roo-akh El-oh-heem) (commonly known as Spirit of God)—The breath of Yahuah moving in creation, empowerment, and prophecy.

Ruach Ha'Qodesh (Roo-akh Ha-ko-desh) (commonly known as The Holy Spirit)—The set-apart Spirit who indwells, convicts, and guides believers.

Selah (Say-lah) (commonly known as Pause and Reflect)—An invitation to pause, ponder, and absorb the weight of revelation.

Sha'ul's (Shah-oolz) (commonly known as Paul's [letters/teachings])—Refers to the epistles of Sha'ul (Paul), grounded in Hebraic thought.

Shalom (Shah-lohm) (commonly known as Peace, Wholeness) — Extends beyond peace—signifying completeness, harmony, and covenant well-being.

The Ruach (The Roo-akh) (commonly known as The Spirit of God)—Describes the very Spirit of Yahuah moving in power and presence.

Yah (Yah) (commonly known as The LORD)—A short form of Yahuah, affirming His covenant Name.

Yahuah — (commonly known as God, LORD, or Jehovah)

Yahusha (Yah-oo-shah) (commonly known as Jesus)—The true Hebrew name of our Savior, meaning "Yahuah is salvation."

Yahusha HaMASHIACH (Messiah) (The Christ) (Yah-oo-shah Ha-mah-shee-akh) (commonly known as Jesus Christ)—The fullness of the Name and title: Yahuah's Anointed Deliverer.

REFERENCES

CHAPTER ONE

Medical News Today

https://www.medicalnewstoday.com › articles › ibd-co...

Dec 22, 2022—A recent study shows that **a common red food dye could cause intestinal inflammation** and trigger inflammatory bowel disease (IBD).

National Institutes of Health (NIH) (.gov)

https://pmc.ncbi.nlm.nih.gov › articles › PMC8266754

by Z He · 2021 · Cited by 79—Here we show that the azo dyes **Red** 40 and Yellow 6, the most abundant **food colorants** in the world, **can** trigger an **IBD**-like **colitis** in mice conditionally ...

Jun 12, 2023—Red Dye 40 is common in: * flavored milk and yogurts. * puddings. * ice cream. * popsicles. * cakes and pastries. * c...

FDA

Cleveland Clinic Health Essentials

Red Dye 40: Side Effects, Foods, Alternatives, & More - GoodRx

Foods that contain Red Dye 40 Many foods that are bright red contain Red Dye 40, including: Breakfast cereals. Sodas and other sof...

GoodRx

Allura Red AC - Wikipedia

When prepared as a lake pigment it is disclosed as Red 40 Lake or Red 40 Aluminum Lake. It is used in some tattoo inks and is used...

Wikipedia

Allura Red AC - an overview | ScienceDirect Topics

Allura red is originally derived from petroleum. It is added into soft drinks, children's medications, and cotton candy. This is t...

ScienceDirect.com

What is Red Dye 40 and What are the Red 40 Alternatives

Jan 16, 2025—The Prevalence of Red Dye 40 in Everyday Products Red dye 40 can be found in a vast range of products, including: Cand...

Tides Commodity Trading Group

Red Dye 40: Safety, Uses, and Food Lists - Everyday Health

Jan 30, 2025—Pastries. Cakes and frosting. Cereals (such as Froot Loops, Lucky Charms, Trix, Fruity Pebbles) Candy and gum (such as...)

Foods with Red Dye 40: Sodas, sports drinks, teas, juices. Sodas and soft drinks are also obvious places where synthetic dyes could be lurking.Packaged snacks, Condiments. Breakfast Cereals. Baking Mixes, Baked Goods, and Pastries.Packaged Fruit Products and Fruit Bars.Country Label Differences & General Risks.

CHAPTER TWO

The Effects of Natural and Synthetic Blue Dyes on Human ...

National Institutes of Health (NIH) (.gov)

https://pmc.ncbi.nlm.nih.gov › articles › PMC8634323

ADDITIONAL EVIDENCE-BASED RESEARCH

Food Additives & Health

- Feingold Association: https://feingold.org/
- Center for Science in the Public Interest (CSPI): https://www.cspinet.org/
- Documentary: *Fed Up* (2014)

History of the Sabbath Change & Church Councils

- "From Sabbath to Sunday" by Samuele Bacchiocchi, Ph.D.

The Catholic Mirror, Sept. 23, 1893 (quotes acknowledging Sunday substitution)

- https://www.sabbathtruth.com/
- "The Two Babylons" by Alexander Hislop
- Encyclopedia Britannica on the Council of Nicaea and the Council of Trent

Name Substitution & Sacred Identity

- "Come Out of Her My People" by C.J. Koster
- Institute for Scripture Research: https://www.isr-messianic.org/
- Ancient Hebrew Research Center: https://www.ancient-hebrew.org/

Social Stratification & Institutional Inequality

- "The New Jim Crow" by Michelle Alexander
- Pew Research: Racial Wealth Gap Data (https://www.pewresearch.org/)

- National Equity Atlas (https://nationalequityatlas.org/)

General Spiritual Discernment

- "Pagan Christianity?" by Frank Viola & George Barna
- Institute for Biblical & Scientific Studies: https://www.bibleandscience.com/
- Blue Letter Bible for original language studies: https://www.blueletterbible.org/
- Food Dyes Health Effects Assessment OEHHA
- Office of Environmental Health Hazard Assessment (.gov)

https://oehha.ca.gov › healthefftsassess041621

Apr 16, 2021—Studies of Blue No. 1 in laboratory animals indicate low absorption ... We found one experimental study of Blue No. 1 GI absorption in.

311 pages

- Red Alert: The Truth About Artificial Red Dye and Their
- Culinary Solvent

https://culinarysolvent.com › blogs › alcohol-for-chefs

Artificial red dye, most commonly Red Dye 40 and Red Dye 3, are petroleum-derived substances used to enhance the visual appeal of foods, drinks, and cosmetics.

www.ingramcontent.com/pod-product-compliance
Lightning Source LLC
Chambersburg PA
CBHW070104080526
44586CB00013B/1185